How You Can Get
BETTER MEDICAL CARE
FOR LESS MONEY

How You Can Get BETTER MEDICAL CARE FOR LESS MONEY

Dr. Morris N. Placere
and
Charles S. Marwick

Walker and Company, New York

First published in the United States of America in 1973 by the Walker Publishing Company, Inc.

Published simultaneously in Canada by Fitzhenry & Whiteside, Limited, Toronto.

ISBN: 0-8027-0387-9

Library of Congress Catalog Card Number: 70-188476

Printed in the United States of America.

10 9 8 7 6 5 4 3 2

CONTENTS

Introduction

WARNING! American medicine may be hazardous to your health.

When you subject yourself to the attentions of a surgeon in the United States today, you stand a chance of being operated upon by a man who may not be properly qualified to do the job. There are statistics to show that half the surgical operations done in American hospitals are performed by men who are not trained for that particular procedure. Furthermore, there are studies that indicate that a great deal of the surgery now performed is unnecessary. There is at work a medical variation of Parkinson's Law: the amount of surgery expands to fill the number of available beds, the operating rooms, and the surgeon's time.

And the problem is not only with surgery. Much the same story can be told about other medical specialties. Many examples will be discussed in this book. They don't make pleasant reading.

Moreover, these types of medical malpractice, which affect the individual patient, also seriously increase the cost of medical care for everyone—for those who need it as well as for those who don't.

In the past fifteen years, the cost of medical care has tripled in the United States. Americans now spend more than $75 billion annually on their medical care—seven percent of the gross national product. Nor does this expenditure show signs of leveling off. Experts predict that by 1975 the U.S. health care bill will be more than $100 billion, and by 1980 well over $150 billion—about 8 percent of the projected gross national product.

The cost of medical care in this country, no matter how it is ultimately financed, is rising out of the reach of all except the most wealthy.

Concern about this skyrocketing cost has led to various proposals—some in the form of bills before Congress—for providing more comprehensive insurance coverage, including forms of national health insurance. These proposals put the cart before the horse. They attempt to deal with the problem of cost by altering the system of payment when what they should be tackling is the problem of quality. None of the proposals under consideration by Congress has any built-in assurance of proper quality control over either physicians or hospitals. Should any of these bills become law, it will merely compound the present problem. If public financing replaces private financing, it will merely encourage the health professionals to continue on their present course. The quality of medicine is going to continue to decline, regardless of the type of financing; a more efficient form of financing may even facilitate the degradation.

We live in a country that has one of the highest ratios in the world of physicians to population, and some of the best-equipped modern hospitals and nursing homes to deliver health care. Yet one segment of the population—the lower socio-economic groups—gets only the most rudimentary attention or none at all under our present health system.

What is not so widely appreciated is that another, even larger segment of the population, the suburban middle class, is over-doctored, medically and surgically. These people receive almost twice the number of operations they need and roughly twice the amount of drugs, along with much unnecessarily prolonged hospitalization and too numerous laboratory tests and X-rays. The underlying reason for this disparity in health care between the poor on one hand and the middle and upper classes on the other is economic. Physicians, hospitals, clinics, the entire gamut of the health industry is geared to supplying medical needs, real or fancied, for those who can afford to pay for them or who have adequate insurance coverage. Those who cannot afford to pay, or cannot get health insurance, or do not have any health insurance at all, are largely neglected.

Thus, the way to improve our health services is not to continue to increase the volume of those services, as most present health plans propose. This is simply pouring money into a bottomless pit. The real need is for more equitable allocation and more intelligent use of our existing medical resources. Both the individual purchaser of medical care and its providers should be discouraged from overusing the various services that make up our health care system, so that the inadequately serviced might be drawn into the system.

The system as it is presently set up in this country encourages over-utilization by the affluent. Physicians, hospitals, and the health insurance industry all play major roles in forcing up the cost of care. In the past ten or fifteen years, the number of hospitals and clinics in the well-to-do suburbs have multiplied rapidly. They have expanded their services and installed a great deal of modern medical equipment, regardless of the real needs of the community for such things. Hospitals have gone in for many hotel-like comforts, television and other frills, on top of these expanded facilities. Unfortunately, this window-dressing is often mistaken by the patient for better medical care.

Having expanded their services, the hospitals that serve the middle class must then seek to encourage the use of these services. Thus, there is continuous pressure to supply more and more tests, more and more surgery, and, in turn, to find more and more patients to fill the new beds. The result is a continuous expansion of use, which in turn leads to increases in cost. All of this is done because there is money to pay for medical care, not because the medical care always is needed.

Like Charlie Chaplin in *Modern Times,* the patient, or consumer of health care, becomes the least important individual in this monstrous health care machine. He has become only a means to an end, the oil to lubricate a fantastic system of *non-health care* that exists for the economic benefit of a vast army of persons, ranging through suppliers of hospital goods, the building construction industry, the health insurance purveyors, the ancillary health personnel, to the nurses and medical and administrative professions—an entire empire that has little relation to the actual health needs of the individual.

The consumer of health care is the victim of this system. He is a pawn in the game of "good health care"—an enormously profitable operation that has fastened itself on him like a leech. The well-to-do American is glutted with health care, while the poor remain largely uncared for.

But you don't have to put up with this type of medical care. There are any number of first rate doctors and surgeons available—if you take the trouble to find them. This book will show you how you can be assured that you're getting good doctors and being treated with reasonable care in reasonable safety.

Most physicians and surgeons are well aware of the incompetence and inefficiency existing within their ranks. For various reasons, they do nothing about it. Since the medical profession is doing little to police itself, it is up to you—the consumer—to blow the whistle on medical incompetents and get them out of the health care business where they have so comfortably embedded themselves at your expense.

You may be playing Russian Roulette with your health—perhaps even your life—unless you know how to check up on your doctor and the whole system of agencies and institutions that purport to help you get better medical care.

How You Can Get
BETTER MEDICAL CARE
FOR LESS MONEY

I

A Tale of Two Patients

Not long ago, an attractive, slim, middle-aged lady whom we'll call Mrs. Barbara S. celebrated a fifth anniversary. It was one of the most important events of her life, for it had been five years since she had been operated on for cancer of the uterus. Mrs. Smith had joined the ever-growing ranks of those who, from the health statisticians' point of view, are regarded as being cured of cancer.

Mrs. S.'s bout with this disease began with a routine annual checkup by her obstetrician, whom she had gone to because he taught at an adjacent medical college. "She seemed in normal health," her doctor recalls today, "but her Pap smear showed a two-plus abnormality and I thought she ought to be studied further."

The Pap smear is a simple test for cancerous cells developed many years ago by a famous New York obstetrician, Dr. George Papanicolau. It involves scraping some cells from the wall of the cervix—the neck of the womb—and then examining them under the microscope to see if there are any abnormal cells present. The extent of the abnormality is

1

reported as a series of plus signs. Negative is normal and the number of plus signs up to five indicates the extent of the abnormality. In Mrs. S.'s case the two-plus abnormality was an indication of the presence of only a marginal degree of malignancy.

"She was 43 years old at the time," her obstetrician observed. "She had two children, a boy and a girl. Her last pregnancy had been ten years before."

Mrs. S. was admitted to a hospital for further study. Under a general anesthetic, her cervix was dilated and a thorough examination made of her uterus and vagina. Further study of the tissues taken at this examination confirmed the original reading of the Pap smear. There were malignant cells in her uterus.

"We could have waited six months to see if the malignancy increased," Mrs. S.'s obstetrician continued, "but frankly, in my experience these two-plus readings are usually signs of early cancer. In view of her age and the fact that she and her husband already had all the children they wanted, I recommended a hysterectomy."

Mrs. S.'s uterus was removed. She recovered completely. In the years since, she has been examined regularly by her obstetrician, and there has been no recurrence of abnormal cells or unusual bleeding. Thanks to modern medical research, the means were available to diagnose the disease early, before it had a chance to spread. Thanks to the intelligence and alertness of her obstetrician she was guided to take the proper course of action. Thanks to careful surgery, the abnormal tissue was removed with the minimum of hazard and disability.

Tragically different was the fate of a young woman of only 22 whom we'll call Mrs. J. When she found herself pregnant, she phoned the hospital nearest to her home and asked for the name of an obstetrician who lived nearby. Because her husband was frequently out of town on business she wanted her baby to be delivered in the nearby hospital, in case of an emergency. She took it for granted that because they lived in a well-to-do suburb that the local hospital would be able to handle something as routine as childbirth.

After an uncomplicated pregnancy, she went into labor and entered the hospital. While delivering the child with the aid of forceps, her obstetrician accidentally tore her vagina and damaged the blood vessels that supply blood to the vagina.

Unable to stop the bleeding, he proceeded to open her abdomen and tied off the major arteries supplying the lower abdomen and legs. This still failed to stop the bleeding. So with the aid of a general surgeon, he removed the uterus. Eventually, they managed to control the bleeding and removed the ligations from the arteries which had by now resulted in stopping the supply of blood to her legs.

Mrs. J., a young woman who had looked forward to raising a happy family, was now unable to have any more children. But far worse was ahead.

Now critically ill and in the intensive care unit, she underwent a tracheotomy by the general surgeon, who also put her into a mechanical respirator to take over her breathing. For six weeks, Mrs. J. breathed air pumped into her lungs by a mechanical respirator. Anyone familiar with the physiology of the lungs could see what was going to happen next.

Mrs. J. developed what is technically known as a tension pneumothorax. This means, literally, air in the chest. In her case, the air had found its way into the chest cavity through a tear in her lung caused by the continuous pumping of air from the respirator at high pressure. Air was leaking out of this rupture in her lung tissue and was getting between the chest wall and the lungs. It built up so much pressure that it now threatened to collapse the lung entirely.

This is an emergency situation. If it went untreated, the heart could be displaced by the increased pressure of air in the chest and this in turn could have interfered with the general circulation of the blood.

To treat this, the general surgeon did a thoractomy—that is, he opened the chest wall with an incision between the ribs to let the air in the chest escape and so allow the lungs to expand again. He did not ask for a specialist in chest surgery to give him any help.

As a result of her first operation (to control the bleeding from the uterus), Mrs. J. had developed a blocked right ureter. (This is the tube that carries the urine from the kidney to the bladder.) She was examined with a cystoscope by a specialist. (A cystoscope is a viewing device inserted into the urinary canal.) A catheter or drainage tube was then pushed into the canal in an attempt to relieve the blockage. This failed, so finally she was re-operated upon. Her right kidney was opened up and drained.

Back in her room and still doggedly fighting for her life, Mrs. J. had another pneumothorax. This time a first-year resident in general surgery did the operation, without any supervision from the first surgeon, who was out to lunch. At no time during these chest operations had any expert in thoracic surgery been consulted.

Mrs. J. now slipped downhill very rapidly. A few days after the second chest operation, she died, having spent more than a month in the intensive care unit of the hospital.

Both of these incidents are true. It is the paradox of American medicine that such incidents happen every day. And don't get the idea that Mrs. S. had been given the benefits of private care in comfortable surroundings and that Mrs. J. was the victim of second-rate "ghetto medicine" in some dark and dreary old-fashioned city hospital. The situation was just the opposite.

Mrs. S. was treated at a major city medical center, a teaching hospital that trains some of this country's best doctors. Mrs. J. on the other hand was in a community hospital just recently expanded to serve a new and relatively wealthy suburban area. Many of the residents in this district are well-educated professional men and women who live in comfortable $100,000 homes.

What happened to Mrs. S. and Mrs. J. illustrates one of the problems of American medical care—both the good and the bad. As Charles Dickens put it in *A Tale of Two Cities:* "It was the best of times, it was the worst of times." In today's American medicine, it is the best of times for the Mrs. S.'s; and at the same time, it is also the worst of times for the Mrs. J.'s.

Within living memory, many of the major diseases that used to plague us have all but vanished. Vaccines have been developed against crippling diseases such as polio and potential killers such as influenza—which in 1919 ended the lives of over 400,000 Americans. It is more than twenty years since a case of smallpox occurred in the United States, and even that one came from abroad.

To be sure, as the old death-dealing diseases have been defeated and their ravages blunted, there has been an increase in the chronic diseases—particularly those associated with older people. Heart disease, for example, accounts for half the deaths in this country, while cancer in all its forms runs second place.

Yet, even among these modern killing diseases, there have been encouraging advances in treatment. Many who would certainly have died as a result of diseased heart valves have had their lives prolonged by having the useless natural valve replaced by an artificial valve. This outstanding advance in surgery has been made only within the past thirteen years. Again, many who might have died from an undue slowing of the pumping action of the heart now continue to live useful lives with a pacemaker, a device permanently implanted in their chest that stimulates the heart artificially. Justice William O. Douglas of the Supreme Court has such a device— just to pull one name out of a very large hatful.

The situation is improving with cancer, too, despite the fear of the disease in the popular mind. The death rate from cancer of the cervix has been cut by half in 25 years. Advances in treatment of other forms of cancer have meant that many people who would have died from the disease 25 or even ten years ago are now living reasonably normal and useful lives. With sophisticated drug therapy, many children who would have died of acute leukemia within a few months are now living to grow up.

Why then, with all this progress—and much more—is so much of medicine held in such low regard by the ordinary man today? Medical costs have tripled in fifteen years and there seems to be no end in sight. Is it irritation over this rapidly increasing cost of obtaining any kind of reasonable medical care? Probably not. People recognize that good medicine is not cheap. They expect to have to pay for good health care as they expect to have to pay for any quality service. The almost universal use of health insurance plans of one type or another is clear evidence of this.

Why are people annoyed with physicians? Because they, as

a professional group, make a lot of money? In this affluent society making a lot of money is a commonplace, and the existence of wealthy purveyors of goods and services in non-medical fields does not raise the hackles of the consumer.

No. The real reason for the disillusion of the medical consumer with the medical profession is his growing realization that too much medical care is incompetently performed, inefficiently administered, often unnecessary, and far too often is poorly controlled. Where there is annoyance over the cost of medical care, it is probably because it is frequently a bad bargain—a cut-rate job at first-rate prices.

As we have seen, in America today one woman can be cured of cancer of the womb while another can go to the hospital to have a normal baby and, through incompetence on the part of medical and surgical staff, end up a corpse. Yet far from being censured or disciplined, the offenders are left free to continue perpetrating their second-rate practices on other unsuspecting patients.

For, while you will hear about the Mrs. S.'s of this world, you will seldom hear about the Mrs. J.'s. Doctors encourage a conspiracy of silence when it comes to discussing their mistakes. As was finally done with Mrs. J., they bury them.

Mistakes can occur in any man's life, and doctors are no exception. To err is human. But to deliberately cover up and support incompetence is criminal. There is a growing feeling among Americans today that there are too many human errors covered up in medicine. They are beginning to come to the conclusion that this spells incompetence.

Although, as we have seen, in many hospitals a woman can be cured of cancer of the womb, not to mention a long list of other serious and potentially lethal diseases, equally there are hospitals where you take your life in your hands when you walk in the door. The problem is how to tell the good from the bad.

It takes time and a little effort to discover where the good medicine is, and then to see that you get it. There is no use expecting doctors to provide good medical care just because they are licensed physicians.

Unfortunately, it is as difficult for the average layman to distinguish between a good or a bad doctor as between a good or a bad hospital. Therefore, it is the responsibility of government health insurers and medical educators to provide guidelines for consumers and to enforce proper control on doctors, hospitals, and nursing homes to insure quality and competence.

II

Charting Your Course
Toward the Right Physician

Your first line of defense, in preventing bad medical care and finding good care, is choosing a good doctor for your family. Nothing can substitute for this. A good doctor who is interested in you is your best protection against incompetent specialists. He'll see to it, in so far as it's humanly possible, that you don't get into the wrong hands. He'll help you get the right treatment when you need it, and, one hopes, he'll also tell you when you don't need treatment—advice you should take.

But don't think that because you already have a good family physician you'll never face the problem of having to find a substitute. We are a footloose society these days. One family in five in the United States moves to a different locality every year. So the chances are that you will, at some point, be faced with finding medical care for yourself and your family in new and unfamiliar surroundings.

It is essential to find a doctor to look after you before you get sick. It is irresponsible to wait until you are ill and then expect to find the best care. When you are actually unwell, possibly in pain, you are in no position to judge the nature of the care you're receiving, and your family is at a disadvantage, for they have no familiar person to discuss your case with to make certain that the care you are getting is appropriate.

So, as soon as you have moved into your new home, start looking for a good family doctor. This will take some shopping around and a good deal of patience. But be a good doctor-shopper by applying the same standards of evaluation to a doctor as you did to buying your house and your car or lining up a suitable school and the many services you use in other walks of life.

Unfortunately, good family doctors are hard to find and getting scarcer. Only about one-fifth of the medical profession in America are general practitioners—the latest name for the GP, by the way, is Family Physician—and many of them, under whatever title they use, are older men. General practitioners are something of a dying breed today.

Let's assume you have to move to another part of the country. Before you leave, ask your present doctor if he knows anyone in your new location. This can frequently turn up useful names that will bear investigation. It will also give you an introduction, since you can use your former doctor as a reference. (Incidentally, if he has found out, through trial and error, some particularly effective form of treatment for whatever tends to ail you, ask him to write a letter describing the problem and the therapy. This can save you a lot of money in needless tests at some future date with a new man. Also, be sure you get copies of all the prescriptions you customarily use. Either your doctor or your pharmacy will supply these.)

If your doctor knows no one in your new location, the

company that the head of your household is now working for probably has a physician who can recommend a neighborhood doctor or specialists such as pediatricians, obstetricians and gynecologists, ear, nose and throat specialists, and the like.

After you've moved, look for a healthy family in your neighborhood and ask them who their doctor is. Don't take the advice of people who seem to have a lot of medical problems! Their judgement on physicians could well be uninformed or even bad.

If you live in or near a city where there is a medical school and a teaching hospital, inquire if they have clinics for private patients. Or call the medical school's department of community medicine, if there is one. Another useful source of information about good local physicians is the chief resident in the particular specialty you want at the nearest medical school. It doesn't matter if you are hundreds of miles from the school, at the other end of the state; this man will almost certainly have formed a useful opinion of the capabilities of the specialist physicians in your area by seeing the patients they have referred to the medical school hospital. Don't expect him to tell you the bad ones, unless he knows you very well, but he will certainly be glad to recommend the good ones. The senior resident (and he is a qualified physician, not a student) in any particular specialty in a good university hospital is by definition practicing the highest standards of medical care himself, supervised by the medical school faculty. Since he is a salaried man, he is relieved of the economic necessity to cut medical corners.

Another handy source of information about the local medical facilities is the public information office at the medical school. They know who the top specialists are.

It is sometimes worthwhile to check with the local medical society and see if they have anyone to whom they can refer you in your own neighborhood. But remember that any names they give you are merely those of physicians who have asked to be listed. You have no guarantee, beyond the fact that a man is a paid-up member of the local medical society, that he is competent.

All right, now you have a few names. The next thing to do is to check them out. For this you need a copy of the *Directory of the American Medical Association,* available in most public libraries. It lists all physicians who are members of the AMA, that is, the majority—about two-thirds—of licensed medical practitioners in the country. Physicians who are not AMA members have recently increased in numbers. It is possible to check on them through the state in which they are licensed to practice, for all physicians are licensed by the state. Membership in the AMA and local medical societies is usually for the doctors' convenience, because it can be helpful to them in their practice and in obtaining hospital privileges. Recently, some medical societies, like those in California and New York, which formerly insisted their members belong to the AMA, have begun to drop this requirement. The result has been a slow but steady decline in MDs who are AMA members.

For the specialists on your list, check the *Directory of Medical Specialists,* also available in most public libraries. All medical school libraries have copies of the *AMA Directory* and the *Directory of Medical Specialists.* The latter is broken down by specialty and then by geographical location. So if, for example, you are checking up on a pediatrician, look first under the pediatrician section, then under the state and city for the name of the man in question.

Now you are ready to begin your comparison shopping.

To save your own time, write up a medical case history of yourself and your children—and be sure you keep a copy of it in your home file! List the illnesses you have had and any operations, then outline your current problems, if any. Describe your symptoms, not what you think is wrong. If you have a letter from your previous doctor, attach it—but make a photocopy of it first! You can leave this with the new doctor, if you decide to stay with him. List the drugs you are taking and note whether you need any prescriptions renewed.

Now you are ready to approach the most promising candidate on your list. Call up his office and ask for an appointment. Explain who you are and why you want to see the doctor, using your former doctor as a reference if it's appropriate.

You may find that this particular doctor is not accepting any more new patients. This is a sign of a good doctor. It shows that he doesn't try to overextend himself by taking on too many people. You can, if you like, ask to be put on his waiting list, if he has one. Meanwhile, go on to the next man on your list.

At this point, before you have even met the doctor you are considering, you should have begun to get some impression of him. The way his office staff handles his phone calls indicates how he feels about his patients—for example, is his secretary brusque? Do you get a busy signal every time you call? Consider what this could mean if you needed a doctor in an emergency. It is perfectly legitimate to ask his office assistant whether it is usually difficult to get an answer on the phone. If she says it is, and if she cannot offer you an appointment in less than six weeks, make it, but then try the next name on your list.

Where some physicians won't take on any more patients than they can handle, there are others who try to serve too many patients. Just as you might find it worthwhile to be treated by the first type, you should avoid the second. It is worth remembering that *the best doctors are not necessarily the busiest.* Indeed, the doctor who is too busy may be the worst doctor for you, no matter how good he is, because it takes time to practice good medicine.

Check how long you have to wait in a doctor's office. If you made a proper appointment and are not being squeezed in at the last minute, you shouldn't have to wait more than twenty minutes. The best way to avoid waiting at all is to make your appointment the doctor's first for the day.

For your initial appointment, as a doctor-shopper, you may have to wait several weeks for an appointment and possibly up to an hour in his waiting room. Because you are a new patient, the doctor is going to want a full medical history. Some of this may be taken by his nurse or she may give you a form to fill out that covers the main points. Here your advance preparation of arming yourself with your own medical history will come in handy.

You still haven't gotten to the doctor yet, but again you're getting an idea of what he is like. Watch his office help as they answer the phone and greet the patients. Are they officious or properly protective of the doctor's time? Are they considerate of those who have to wait? Your doctor's assistant can be your best friend in an emergency, so be prepared to get on the right side of these polite though often infuriating people. On the other hand, don't let them push you around or brush you off. The good doctor's staff reflects his own approach to his patients, so observe them. It could be a profitable hour.

When you eventually get in to see the doctor, remind him why you're there. Don't be backward about bringing up such pertinent questions as fees, the usual length of time it takes to get to see him, how he handles emergency calls, and what his affiliations are with the local hospitals. Ask if he makes house calls, but don't worry too much if he says he doesn't. You can do a lot on the telephone these days.

The physicians' magazine, *Medical Economics*—a publication largely devoted to informing doctors on the most efficient way to run their practice—once printed a letter from a physician complaining about prospective patients who came to his office, taking up his time, asking awkward questions about his training, his fees, and other aspects of the way he organized his practice.

"Answering their questions can be embarrassing," he wrote. "What should I do about such doctor-shoppers?"

Wisely, the magazine recommended that he try to answer such individuals' questions as fully and frankly as possible. It pointed out that people smart enough to try to find out what they were buying in the way of a physician were more likely to end up better patients.

The good doctor will be interested in you as a person, not simply as another case. He will imperceptibly draw you out, so that you will tell him what is really on your mind. He will take the trouble to learn your name and pronounce it correctly, and he will show some awareness of your particular situation and problem, even if it is just loneliness in a new and strange town.

After you have left his office, think back and ask yourself: "Did the doctor try to find out about me as a person, or was he too busy selling himself and his importance, or subtly finding out how much money I made?"

Beyond a point, the best doctor for you is one whose personality and approach suits yours. Some people prefer a doctor who is all business. Others want someone who indicates some humanity. This has little to do with medical competence, but these are important elements nevertheless. If you don't like someone, you cannot trust them, and if you cannot trust your doctor, he cannot give you the best medical care.

Remember, too, that you may need to depend on this doctor in a crisis. Does he seem capable of handling it—and you? Good doctors know that patients shop for their medical services, and they appreciate this. If you choose a man and go back to him, you are likely to be treated with respect for your intelligence.

What about annual medical checkups? In other words, apart from actual bouts of illness, how often should you see your doctor? Are checkups really a useful way to catch sickness before it becomes a major problem?

There is no doubt that checkups play a useful role in preventive medicine but if you are normal and healthy, during most of your lifetime, it is not really necessary to have a checkup every year. Here is our prescription.

A woman should be under the care of her doctor during pregnancy. Regular prenatal care is helpful in making sure that the baby develops normally and in spotting any potential difficulties that may occur at birth. The baby will be examined when it is born, and when it is ready to be discharged from the hospital, it should have a checkup. After the first year of life, the normal infant will be ready for most routine immunizations—he or she may have already had some shots at six months.

A child should be examined on entering nursery school or kindergarten, again during his grade school years, and on entering high school and college. He will of course get a medical examination if he enters the military service, and both sexes often have to pass physical examinations before starting work in large corporations. A medical checkup is in order at the time of marriage, apart from the mandatory blood tests for venereal disease that most states require for a marriage license.

But as long as you are healthy, a regular checkup should not be necessary until about the age of 40. After that, you might want to see your doctor approximately every two to three years until you are in your fifties. For the next ten years, you might consider an annual checkup, but after you reach 65 or 70, you can cut this down and go back to see your doctor every two to three years, unless, of course, there is any serious abnormality that should be watched.

At the risk of repetition, let us emphasize that as long as you remain in good general health, there is no point in worrying about minor abnormalities as you grow older. These are probably to be expected. Quite often you can do more harm than good if you insist that your doctor try to correct them (or you let him talk you into trying). For example, the sugar levels of a person's blood rise normally with age, and although some doctors have thought that this might be a sign of impending diabetes and would try to reduce the sugar levels in older patients nearer to what they regarded as normal, most physicians today would be less likely to be concerned with bringing an elderly patient's sugar levels down to those of a forty-year-old.

This dynamic view of the medical checkups you need during your lifetime is more realistic, in terms of both the cost of such services and the realities of health, than is the automatic annual checkup, regardless of what is found (or not found). The British, for example, do not recommend taking a Pap smear from a normal patient more often than once every three years. They have found that, while this will not uncover every last case of cervical cancer, it does spot the majority of them, and in good time. As we gain experience, similar data are being gathered on other screening tests. So, if you use your doctor and the services he has available with intelligence, you can expect to receive the maximum benefit with the minimum of risk—and expense.

For what is known as primary care, the ideal man to have as a family doctor is a good general practitioner. But unfortunately, as we have seen, they are in short supply today. So you may have to go to an internist, that is, a specialist in internal medicine, who is, for most practical purposes, the next best thing as a substitute for a GP. Internists are popularly known as the rich man's GP, because being specialists, they can charge more per visit. Make sure, if you use an internist, that he is in fact qualified, by looking him up in the *Directory of Medical Specialists*. If he is not a board-certified internist and he charges specialists' fees, ask him bluntly why he does so. Make him justify the extra expense to you, and if he refuses to do so, be wary of his recommendations from then on.

It's important in health care to have a good all-round man as your primary physician. It is better if he is not a specialist. Specialists are necessary, but they tend to view a patient's problem through their own specialist spectacles. If they are surgeons, surgery is more likely to be recommended as the answer to your problem. If they are gastroenterologists, they'll tend to find the sources of your problem in the abdomen. Nor does it help if you yourself try to decide what specialist you ought to see. It may seem sensible, if you have a pain in your chest, to go to a chest specialist. But in reality, the cause of this pain may have nothing to do with the thoracic region.

If you have children, think carefully before sending them to a pediatrician. If they are normal and healthy, this may be unnecessary and simply involve you in needless expense. A family doctor can just as easily give routine immunization shots and see them through routine childhood illnesses. Reflect for a moment how much attention some of those busy pediatricians can actually provide. Some see as many as a hundred children a day. Under these circumstances, how can the care they deliver be worth a specialist's fee?

One type of specialist who is becoming increasingly involved in primary care services is, oddly enough, the surgeon. One reason is that there isn't enough surgery to keep him busy, so he has been moving in on the generalist and seeing patients directly. This finding emerged from a survey made by Dr. John Stubbs, himself a general surgeon, while he was at the Sloan School of Management at the Massachusetts Institute of Technology. He found that most of the surgical patients he interviewed looked to their surgeon for primary medical care.

What Dr. Stubbs has to say about choosing a surgeon as your family physician should make you very wary.

"When specialists such as surgeons provide primary care, the whole balance and rational structure of the medical team is distorted," he notes. "The specialist is now in competition with the generalist for primary care patients. Under these circumstances, it is only natural that the generalist is less willing to refer his problem patients. He is less inclined to seek consultation from his competitor. At best this reticence merely reduces the productivity of the generalist and prolongs the patient's discomfort. At worst, it may cost the patient his life."

Remember, Dr. Stubbs is talking about you.

Obtaining good medical services is probably going to become easier in the future. Compared with the present generation of physicians, the younger generation of doctors seems interested in getting back to family practice or community medicine and to be keeping an open mind on health programs and insurance plans.

This trend—and it is still just that—may not come to anything nor will it occur overnight. But the chances are real that change will come from within the profession as well as from outside.

Not only you, the patient, have been dissatisfied with the way medical services have been provided; many members of the medical profession have been unhappy too. In their view, failure to change the system has interfered with their mission in life, which is the provision of service to their patients.

III

An Apple a Day

The best way to keep your medical bills down, unquestionably, is to stay healthy. That way you avoid the need for going to your doctor at all, except for routine checkups.

Fortunately, despite all the popular talk about dread diseases of one type or another, a state of good health is far more prevalent than one of sickness. The very word disease (dis-ease) indicates as much. And even if you do get sick, the chances are that you will get better, regardless of what a doctor does—or does not—do.

However, if you really sense that you are unwell, you should check with your doctor. But exercise some discrimination about when you call him and how you do it. These days, he may bill you for the telephone advice, which is fair enough because he is doing you a service. Many doctors today have a reduced scale of fees for telephone consultations.

So the first step in keeping medical bills down is resisting the temptation to call your doctor every time you have an ache or sniffle. And if you do feel it is necessary to get in

21

touch with him, see if a telephone conversation won't do the trick. Take your temperature and make some penciled notes of your symptoms before you pick up the phone. Perhaps all you need is a mild tranquilizer or something to help you rest while your body is fighting off the illness.

Good doctors appreciate patients who use their services intelligently. You put them on your side when you show that you realize this. Like the boy who cried "Wolf!" there comes a point when, if you run to your doctor every time something seems wrong, he won't pay much attention when you really need him. So don't claim it's an emergency every time you phone and his secretary says, "He's out of the office."

All well and good, you may say, but what do I do when I'm really faced with sickness? Here's a common example. You have come down with what you suspect is the flu that's going around. If you are reasonably healthy and have no history of respiratory or heart disease, you should recover without any difficulty. There is an old medical saying that "a cold runs its course in a fortnight if you don't see a doctor, and fourteen days if you have treatment for it."

But be sensible. Don't go to work or attend the football game as if nothing were wrong. Stay home and in bed if you have a fever or don't feel like getting up and dressed. Often an illness is the body's plea for rest. So nurse yourself, and don't get chilled. Normally there is no need to go and see your doctor—and almost certainly he will not come to see *you*. There is usually nothing he can do for you that the natural disease-fighting machinery in your body is not already doing. You could make yourself worse going out to his office and sitting in his waiting room for an hour, possibly infecting other patients or even picking up fresh infection yourself.

Influenza, like the common cold, is a virus disease, and as yet, medicine has no readily available therapy that will combat a virus the way antibiotics fight bacteria. Some anti-viral drugs are now being developed, but their use is still limited. This is because in order to kill the viral infection, they have to interfere with the body's normal cell mechanism, its metabolism. The only way viruses can multiply in the body is within the cell itself, so to be successful, anti-viral drugs must interfere with the cell's normal activity, which can be hazardous. Thus, use of these drugs is seldom justifiable for the majority of everyday virus diseases such as flu and colds.

So when you have a virus disease, all your doctor can do is help you through the acute—and often miserable—stage of the infection by prescribing such simple drugs as aspirin or a decongestant. Unless you have some secondary complication, like a lung infection, you should resist taking antibiotics. Indeed if your doctor prescribes an antibiotic for you when you have flu, you should ask him why he is prescribing it. This applies equally to any other prescription drug he recommends. For more advice on taking drugs see Chapter IV, on their use and abuse.

For normally healthy people, the ordinary ailments in most instances are not serious. Nor is there anything complicated about keeping healthy. It involves two simple principles, one positive and the other negative. The positive principle is to cultivate good health; the negative one is to avoid known hazards to your health.

Under the first category come such matters as taking plenty of exercise and eating sensibly. Under the second are such equally obvious measures as not smoking, drinking, or pushing yourself to excess. Rather mundane, not very exciting, you say. Agreed. There is no grand, royal road to health. The condition is achieved mostly through common sense.

Nor is this road a one-way street. Quite apart from making sure your doctor doesn't prescribe unnecessary medication or recommend unneeded treatment, make sure that you, in turn, do not demand procedures or drugs that your doctor says are not necessary. Tonsillectomies are a good example. It is widely agreed by the best surgeons and pediatricians that the majority of such operations are unnecessary. So don't compound this situation by demanding that your Tommy have his tonsils out just because all the other children on the block have had theirs out. Keeping up with the Joneses may help build your ego, but don't make your children pay the price. And if your doctor says your child should have his tonsils out, double check with an independent specialist first. A tonsillectomy, like any surgery, carries a definite risk. Make sure this risk is worth taking.

Perhaps because the maintenance of health is not exciting stuff, particularly for the medical profession, doctors call it preventive medicine or public health and tend to dismiss the patient's efforts to stay well as not too important. This is not entirely the doctor's fault—it is how he has been conditioned to think. Indeed this is one of the problems of modern medicine. In medical schools students are taught how to treat diseases. This, they are told, is the big challenge—the diagnosis and successful handling of disorders with its logical sequel, the dramatic surgical repair of diseased or injured bodies. Only in very rare instances are medical students reminded that it is not diseases but patients to whom they must devote most attention.

Unfortunately, for reasons that are beyond the scope of consideration in this book, medical schools and medical education in the U.S. has in the past quarter of a century devoted more and more attention to the science of medicine—diagnosis and treatment of disease—and less to the art or human side of medicine.

The result is that an entire generation of physicians has grown up familiar with all the modern scientific tools of diagnosis and treatment but with too little knowledge of or concern for the individual who happens to have the disease. Indeed, this scientific attitude toward medicine has even been incorporated into what is perhaps the least scientific of all the medical specialties—psychiatry—with results that are little short of disastrous.

Doctors are not alone in this way of thinking. It is an expression of how modern man deals with the problems of his society. We are all science oriented and more at home with what we think are scientific elucidations and solutions to problems than we are with non-scientific ones. We verbalize our problems and solutions in scientific terms often without realizing that by so doing we are merely clouding the issues, not clarifying them. Physicians are part of our society and quite apart from the way they are trained, they of necessity act as we all do. In other words, they tend to give impressive names to ordinary diseases. No one for example ever seems to have a common cold these days—it is always either a virus or an "upper respiratory infection."

There are many popular books on how to stay well and keep fit. Read some of them. Just remember that not all their advice should be taken too literally. Good health does not lie in imbibing a specially-made brew, adhering to some esoteric spartan regimen, or eating only honey produced by bees at midsummer. However, such books often contain much good advice which, when filtered through your own knowledge of how you and your family live, can help you keep well and, above all, keep your doctor at bay!

Preventing the onset of disease is ninety percent of the battle. No matter how good your doctor is, no matter how efficient modern medicine and surgery may be, treating an illness once it has started is never as satisfactory as preventing it in the first place. In light of this, it becomes difficult to understand the popularity of heart transplant surgery. Even if the operation ever becomes truly therapeutic (and that day is far off) such surgery can never be as good as keeping the heart that you've got in good shape. If you don't believe this, ask the next person you meet who wears artificial teeth whether he thinks they're better than the ones he had originally.

How effectively prevention can work is well illustrated by the experiences of the medical officer of a commercial airline. This doctor has developed a method of spotting impending heart disease in the pilots under his care. More practically, he has devised an exercise regimen for these individuals. Basically, it consists of graduated amounts of brisk walking, from a mile or so to three or four miles every day.

Of the pilots who have taken his advice and done the exercises, a smaller percentage have been grounded for heart abnormalities than those who disregarded the regimen. Pilots, of course, have a strong inducement to keep healthy because if they don't meet basic health requirements they don't have their pilot's licenses renewed. This can mean considerable loss of income.

Well, you may say, but I'm not an airline pilot. Just think for a minute, though. Even if you are unlikely to be relegated to some lower-paying, less interesting job because of a physical ailment, it will still reward you to devote some attention to physical fitness. After all, if you do develop a chronic disease, it means a loss in income, for you will then have to spend some of your hard-earned money for doctors' care and drugs. Your insurance is unlikely to cover it all, as you will see in Chapter XIII, on health insurance. It is also conceivable that you may be overlooked for promotion in your company because your health is unreliable. This is true both for men and for women—particularly for the so-called weaker sex.

"It is more advisable to pass a careful physical examination if one intends to be sedentary—in order to establish whether one's health can stand the inactivity" says Dr. Samuel M. Fox III, a prominent cardiologist. So get some exercise, regularly every day—real exercise, not just a round of golf or a tennis game once a week in the nice weather. And if you do play golf, walk the course. Don't ride around it in one of those carts. Perhaps the best exercise in the world is walking. We know a physician, an anesthesiologist, who deliberately lives within walking distance of the hospital where he works. When he gets a call for his services, even as often happens in the middle of the night, all he has to do is dress and walk. The exercise stimulates his mind and by the time he has reached the hospital he is fully alert. Not only that, but his wife does her daily shopping on foot and his four children walk to school. This family lives in a midwestern city and they have gone to considerable trouble to accomplish this, moving several times to different areas, but they feel it has been well worth it.

This may sound like too drastic a change in the way most of us live. But more and more, sensible people are beginning to act on such ideas today. Witness, for example, the growing popularity of yoga. This is an excellent way to keep fit, since yoga is not just calisthenics, it is training for the mind as well as the body, and the exercises have a real effect on the body's physiology over and above muscle toning. Yoga trains you to think yourself healthy. Together with swimming and other good forms of exercise, yoga classes may be found these days at your nearest "Y."

Diet is another case in point. It is far easier to avoid putting on weight than to get it off once it is there. A minute in the mouth, it has been said, can mean a lifetime on the hips. Proper eating habits that ensure good nutrition without building surplus fat should be encouraged on a family rather than on just an individual basis. If one family member is too heavy, the chances are that the others have the same potential—in any event, it will do them no harm to cut out the calorie-laden sauces and desserts. According to recent statistics 60,000,000 Americans know they are overweight.

Again, common sense is your guide. Almost every newspaper or magazine contains information on what constitutes good diet, and there is increasing emphasis among the purveyors of foodstuffs to make the consumer aware of the contents of packaged or canned foods. So there is no excuse today for anyone not to know what—or how much—he or she should eat.

Besides such positive steps to ensure good health, you can also take action to sidestep health hazards. We have already mentioned excessive smoking and drinking as two obvious habits to avoid if you wish to stay healthy. The nonsmoker's risk of disease is considerably reduced by comparison with that of the smoker, not only in relation to serious problems like cancer, emphysema, or heart disease, but also in the daily miseries of sore throats and inflamed sinuses. This has been convincingly demonstrated by many studies done over the past quarter of a century.

There are many other aspects of our modern life where, with a little thought and planning, you can reduce risks to your health. One excellent instance is using public transportation instead of commuting by automobile. The risk of injury or death in a private car is much higher than in a train or bus. In 1970, there were 55,000 deaths from automobile accidents in the U.S. and, more important from our point of view, there were 2,000,000 injuries on the roads severe enough to involve a stay of more than one day in the hospital. By reducing the mileage you drive, you also reduce your chances of being injured in a road accident. This is particularly important for the daily drive to and from work. At the end of the day you are probably tired and unable to react with sufficient speed to assure safety on modern, high-speed highways. If you are caught in traffic jams, the situation can be even worse, because the build-up of carbon monoxide in the surrounding air can further slow your mental alertness. Moreover, the block or two that you walk to the bus or train gives you at least a minimum amount of exercise and fresh air daily.

We have allowed our familiarity with the automobile to lull us into a feeling that driving a car requires no more than casual attention. But driving is work—hard, tense work— and to stay alive on the roads you need every faculty functioning at key pitch.

So sit down and consider your way of life objectively and you will easily find many ways to reduce hazards to health in your daily program, whether at work, at play, or at home. For instance, most accidents happen in a person's own house. All too many of these are the result of carelessness in noticing a loose step, a shaky ladder, a slippery floor, inflammable fabrics or objects lying around. Not only children and the elderly are endangered—one youngish woman spent four years between crutches and a wheelchair because she tripped over a pile of carpeting in her summer cottage.

As for safety outside the home, it is not suggested that you never venture out onto the road or engage in safe sports. Life is full of risks. We take chances whenever we cross the street, but we calculate them. We wait for the traffic light to bring vehicles to a halt so we can cross at the intersection with the minimum risk of being hit. As the statisticians put it, the benefit-to-risk ratio at such times is high.

A recent example of this benefit-to-risk ratio comes from medical practice: smallpox vaccination. There is a slight risk that a child can become seriously ill or even die from a smallpox vaccination. In 1971, the U.S. Public Health Service decided this risk was greater than the risk children ran today of contracting the disease, so they recommended that public health authorities and physicians discontinue the routine practice of vaccinating young children against smallpox. This decision was made in the light of the knowledge that smallpox is a disappearing disease today, throughout the world, and the chance of anyone contracting it in America is negligible. Fifty or even twenty-five years ago, the risk from the vaccination would have been worthwhile because there was still a chance of being exposed to smallpox. Incidentally, public health authorities still recommend smallpox vaccination for those who travel to countries where the disease has not yet been eradicated. It is also vitally important that children continue to be immunized against prevalent childhood diseases.

The point is, there are many things in our daily life that could be injurious to health. Avoid them when you reasonably can. Where you cannot, or do not want to, then try to estimate the risk involved. With this knowledge, you may be able to minimize this risk and so obtain the maximum benefit. Don't give up things you genuinely enjoy on the remote chance that they might harm you. For instance, although you could break a leg, skiing is a healthier way to spend a winter weekend than sitting around indoors considering your health and feeling bored—a sure way to think yourself sick.

Let us conclude this chapter with a case report published some years ago in the *British Medical Journal* by a well-known British physician, Dr. Richard Asher. "Many cases of unusual illnesses are described in these columns," Dr. Asher wrote, "so it may make a change if I report a case of unusual health.

"Fanny, as everyone calls her, is now 90 years of age. She works as cook and general servant at a girls' day school in London. She left school at the age of thirteen and started work in domestic service. Since then she has worked at this profession without any illness or absence from work except for ten days in 1932 when she had bronchitis and severe fatigue after nursing her husband, who had a fatal illness.

"She started her present post 42 years ago; it is both strenuous and responsible. She cooks for 90 people and is also housekeeper to the headmistress. She is an alert, spry little woman who moves quickly and vigorously. She enjoys her work, and her mistress, who is devoted to her, regards her as a treasure.

"My knowledge of her," concluded Dr. Asher, "is purely social; she never consults doctors. 'I don't believe in them,' she says."

IV

Common Sense on Using Drugs

Scene: Nurses' station in a hospital.

A physician is talking to a boy's father: "I'm going to try your son on a course of chloramphenicol. That bone infection is not responding to other antibiotics. It's either that or surgery."

"I suppose so," the father replies, but, because he is a medical writer, he adds, "Don't you think you ought to keep an eye on his blood cells while he's being treated?"

"Oh, I don't think that's necessary," his physician answers, "just for the short period that he'll be under treatment. We'll know very quickly whether the infection is going to respond."

But the boy's father persisted. And after looking up the recommendations on the use of this drug (which pointed out the need for extreme caution), the physician finally agreed to keep an eye on the boy's blood cells.

Scene: A doctor's office. Patient, a middle-aged housewife, is talking:

"Doctor, I saw an article in the newspaper the other day

33

that said that this drug you prescribed for me to control TB could cause damage to the liver. And patients who were taking this drug should be watched for signs of liver damage. So, don't you think . . . "

"Don't believe anything you read in the papers about medicine," her doctor told her.

Scene: Another doctor's office.

It was the sixth visit that month for Mrs. Jones. Her doctor sighed as she came through the door. Automatically, he reached for his prescription pad. And as he listened to her lengthy account of her complaints, he began writing out a prescription for a tranquilizer she had not yet tried. As soon as he decently could, he ushered her out, prescription in hand.

We hear a lot about drug abuse these days—kids getting busted for possessing "pot," for example. But one major area of drug abuse is entirely outside the purview of present laws. It is the entirely legal but highly unintelligent use of therapeutically useful agents by physicians and their patients. This abuse originates in ignorance, carelessness, or laziness.

The Food and Drug Administration estimates that half a billion dollars a year is spent on drugs in the United States that have no valid proof of efficacy. This figure does not include the misuse of legitimate agents. Not long ago, a doctor wrote a letter to the *New England Journal of Medicine* describing a patient who consumed 20 different drugs a day— a total of 94 pills. These pills were all for different symptoms or to counteract the side effects caused by the drugs taken for these symptoms. Many drugs that exercise a therapeutic effect also have undesirable side effects, which in turn need additional drugs to keep them in control.

Take our three little vignettes—all taken from real life, just as they happened. In the first case, the doctor—any doctor—should have known that chloramphenicol carries a serious risk of severely damaging the blood cells, and he should have considered taking the necessary precautions to watch for this damage without having to be prompted by the boy's family.

In the second case, no matter what a physician may think of popular newspaper stories about drug hazards, he should have taken the trouble to find out whether the anti-TB drug that his patient was on was doing any damage to her liver. If he had read the newspaper article, which he so brusquely scorned, he would have known of the existence of a report on the problem by public health officials and he could have gotten a copy of it.

Finally, in the third case, we're almost on the doctor's side. Mrs. Jones had been pestering her physician for weeks. There was nothing organically wrong with her, yet she insisted on getting a prescription for drugs that, more likely than not, were doing nothing for her except costing money. The fault here lay in her doctor's placidly going along with her and not taking a few minutes to educate his patient about her health. Possibly if he had also devoted a little time— once at any rate—to try to find out what was at the root of her drug taking, what problem was on her mind, he might have found that a few kindly words of advice would have worked as well as the tranquilizers. And she wouldn't have been back the following week.

Drugs today are far more potent and therapeutically useful than they were even thirty years ago. Therein lies the problem with them. To be effective means by definition that a drug may be toxic. If it were not, it would do no good. This means that you, the patient, should take drugs only when you need them, not just whenever you think you might need them. You should also find out something about drugs in general, and above all, when your doctor prescribes a drug for you, you should ask him why he is prescribing it, how frequently he wants you to take it and for how long. It is up to the physician to tell the pharmacist to put the name of the drug and the dosage prescribed on the label. He should also add some description of what the drug is to be used for, i.e., as a sleeping pill, for headaches, diabetes, high blood pressure, or whatever. Make sure that your doctor does this because it is not the pharmacist's responsibility.

Mistakes can happen all too easily. One lady taking anticoagulant drugs very nearly died from excessive bleeding because the instructions on her bottle of pills were incorrectly typed out by the pharmacist. She had not understood what her doctor had told her, and she simply followed the instructions on the label. Fortunately, her son, a physician in another city, had the habit of phoning her every weekend—and this saved her life. As he always did, he asked about her medicines and in this case found that she was taking four times the needed amount of a common anticoagulant. He told his mother to stop it immediately, then dialed her doctor, repeated their conversation, and got the situation straightened out.

Because drugs play such an important part in today's medicine, it is vital to have some knowledge of them. Drugs fall into two main divisions—proprietary drugs and prescription drugs. The first type—which include such examples as aspirin, antacid pills, and most cold remedies—can be bought over the counter at your local drug store without a prescription. To obtain the second class, however, you must have a doctor's prescription—hence the name prescription drug.

It is one of the peculiar quirks of medicine that physicians are often quite unaware of the cost of the many things they order for their patients. Drugs are no exception. In a particular situation, a physician may tend to prescribe a drug he has heard a lot about. Its cost is unlikely to concern him. After all, he isn't buying it himself.

Doctors are bombarded by drug manufacturers with advertising and promotional material on drugs for treating some particular condition. When a physician sees a patient with that condition, he almost automatically prescribes the drug he has heard and read about. Of course, his own experience and possibly that of physician friends has led him to conclude that the drug in question is as reliable a product as such things can be for the condition he is faced with. But very often he does not know that there are other drugs which, on investigation, might be just as good for the problem and also much cheaper.

Many trade-name drugs have what are called generic equivalents. A generic drug is one whose patent or copyright has run out. A company that develops a drug can and usually does take out a patent on it, providing it is unique. This patent (not to be confused with an old-style patent medicine) lasts for years and in that time no one else may manufacture that drug without the patent owner's permission. But after the patent has run out, any firm can make and market this drug because it is then a generic product. If you are going to be on a drug for any length of time, query your doctor about taking the generic equivalent, if it exists, because often it is much cheaper than a name brand and has the same therapeutic effect.

When you are discussing this drug with your doctor, have him look it up in a publication called PDR, which stands for *Physicians' Desk Reference.* This book carries a listing of most common prescription drugs along with full instructions on how they are to be used, including warnings and precautions connected with their use.

Since modern drugs to be effective must necessarily be toxic, they must be taken with care and with some appreciation of their hazards. So it's a good idea to get a copy of the information that your doctor has in his PDR. Fortunately, this information is easily obtainable. When you are at the drugstore ordering your prescription, ask your pharmacist for a copy of the labeling for that particular drug. This labeling—which, incidentally, is not simply the label on the bottle you receive—carries the full chemical description of the drug, how it is to be used, and the hazards, if any, involved in its use. The labeling is drafted by the manufacturer of the drug and must be approved by the Food and Drug Administration before the drug can be licensed. It's usually somewhat heavy reading, but a study of it could be rewarding—perhaps even lifesaving.

Needless to say, make sure that your prescription is a reasonable one under the circumstances of your taking the drug. If you are to take a pill three times a day for a week, make sure you only get 21 pills, not 24 or 28. Cheaper by the dozen is no bargain in any business, least of all in drug therapy, if you don't need the item.

Don't keep old drugs around, especially prescription drugs. If you don't need a drug, don't have it in the house. It may be swallowed by mistake or children may get at it.

If your doctor thinks you should have the more expensive

trade-name drug rather than the cheaper generic product, make sure that your pharmacist doesn't pull a fast one on you by switching to the generic drug, then charging you for the trade-name variety. It's been done. If you're suspicious, call your doctor and read him the name imprinted on the pills, or take them to his office and show them to him.

Pharmacists charge widely varying markups for their services. Apart from the list price of the drug (that is, what it costs the pharmacist) you may find that one store's handling charge, or retail price, may be several times higher than that of another's. This could be reasonable. Some drug stores keep large inventories on hand, which can mean better service. But it also costs money. Other drug stores may be paying high rents or carrying high insurance costs. All these things affect the pharmacists' cost of doing business, and this cost is passed on to you. So shop around for a good pharmacy just as you would for any other kind of retail outlet.

However, inexpensive drugs are not all necessarily bargains. Some fly-by-night manufacturers turn out pills that contain less than the specified amount of the active ingredient. There have been instances when they have even stamped the name of the manufacturer of the genuine product on the pill or the capsule. Of course, this is illegal and the law usually catches up with such people eventually, but in the meantime you may have been victimized. This is a good reason for dealing with a reputable pharmacist, and it is also why your doctor may hesitate to change from a product that he knows from experience to be reliable. (A good doctor can refer you to a reliable drug store if you are new to the neighborhood.)

Here's another money-saving tip if you're taking drugs for some chronic condition like high blood pressure or diabetes.

From time to time your prescription for these agents will need to be renewed and your doctor may ask you to come in to see him before he renews it. On this visit, make sure that he does something for you that you need. If all he does is write out a prescription for another three months' worth of pills, you've wasted your money and your time and, incidentally, your doctor's time as well.

A good doctor can have his office phone your pharmacy and renew your prescription (or give you a new one) without your coming in for an office visit. However, he may really need to see you periodically when you are on long-term drug treatment, even if everything seems all right to you. Just make sure that he makes some use of your presence, such as taking a blood sample, and does not simply use you as a messenger to take your renewed prescription to the pharmacist—a service for which of course you will be billed by your doctor.

Drugs today are becoming more and more sophisticated and powerful in their action, although there are greater benefits to be gained from these modern drugs so also there are greater risks in using them. A good principle, therefore, is never to take any drug unless you need it.

Sometimes the untoward effects of drugs can lie hidden for many years, and ignorance of their side effects cannot always be blamed on the manufacturer or the doctor. Recently, three Boston physicians found that a drug used to prevent miscarriages seemed to be associated with vaginal cancer twenty years later. And this cancer did not occur in the women who had been given the drug but in the female offspring they had been carrying while they were taking it!

The possible hazards of a drug are frequently difficult to pin down, and you cannot expect the manufacturer or even the Food and Drug Administration to uncover all of them. Sometimes, indeed, skilled pharmacological scientists don't know that there may be a hazard. Thus you have a right to be skeptical of the busy medical practitioner whose knowledge of pharmaceutical chemistry is probably limited to a few lectures at medical school plus what the manufacturers see fit to tell him.

Another point you should appreciate about all drugs is that the same agent taken by one individual may not work in the same way—and perhaps not even at all—when it is taken by another. This means that no one can be absolutely sure that you will not have an untoward reaction from a drug or that when you are given a drug it will do its job. This may have nothing to do with lack of skill on the part of your doctor or with inferior drugs or even a failure by the government licensing agency.

Even with correct dosage and proper methods of use, a drug can still fail to do the job or can cause toxic reactions. The human body is not a predictable contrivance, like an automobile, which can be tuned up to some set standard. We are all different, and none of us function in precisely the same manner.

The effectiveness of biological agents and drugs is determined by the limits of biological probability. An agent may be over 90 percent effective in any one group of patients, but that doesn't help you if you are in the other 5 or 8 percent.

Nothing in biology or medicine is 100 percent. And particularly in the drug field it is true that one man's meat can be another man's poison.

V

The Modern Body Snatchers

For years, young Mrs. Sylvia G., at one time an attractive, vivacious blond, had been living on predigested baby foods because she could swallow only with the greatest difficulty. She was losing weight steadily, her cheeks had become sunken; she looked far older than her 30 years. She was under the care of an internist whom she had gone to regularly, but she had obtained no relief through his treatment.

Her physician had diagnosed her condition as scleroderma of the esophagus. Scleroderma is characterized by a stiffening and thickening of the skin. It can also affect the digestive tract, as Mrs. G's internist maintained it had. In such cases this condition can cause death from starvation, since it can prevent food from being swallowed, or, if swallowed, from being satisfactorily absorbed by the intestines. There is no completely satisfactory treatment for scleroderma.

Finally, out of sheer desperation and on her own initiative, Mrs. G. decided to consult a thoracic surgical specialist, since she had heard he had been able to help some other people in the community who could not swallow food normally.

This surgeon found that her problem was caused by a functional stricture, or narrowing, of the esophagus at the point where it enters the stomach. The condition is known technically as achalasia. In Mrs. G.'s case, it was easily treated by surgery, and she obtained immediate relief after the operation. In fact, she was enjoying normal foods— including a steak—before she was even discharged from the hospital. She rapidly regained weight and has since lived a normal, happy life, eating whatever she wants.

Fifty-eight-year-old William R. had suffered from shortness of breath for years. For the past three years, he had been treated for chronic lung disease and been declared totally disabled by his general practitioner and by an internist who was head of the department of medicine at the local hospital in the suburban community where he lived. Mr. R.'s son was studying at an adjacent medical center, and he insisted that his father see a specialist there.

The true cause of Mr. R.'s problem was then uncovered. Careful examination revealed a loud murmur in his heart and cardiac catheterization revealed an abnormal blood vessel connecting the blood supply between the artery that sends blood from the heart to the lungs, where it receives oxygen. During fetal life, this connection is necessary, since the lungs are not used to oxygenate the blood while the baby is still in its mother's womb. But after birth, this connection normally closes down. In Mr. R.'s case, it had never closed properly, so his oxygenated blood was being diluted with non-oxygenated blood. Therefore, he experienced shortness of breath, as well as other related problems.

Fortunately, it is a simple matter, relatively, to operate on the chest and tie off this abnormal blood vessel. Indeed, this was the essential feature of the first operation to successfully cure a congenital defect of the heart and associated blood vessels. It was performed by Dr. Robert E. Gross of the Harvard Medical School in 1938, on a seven-year-old girl at the Children's Hospital in Boston. The operation marked the real beginning of surgery on the heart and the great vessels, surgery that is now so common.

Mr. R.'s specialist recommended this surgery. But the internist who had been treating him did not agree with this recommendation and declined his approval for the operation. At his family's insistence, however, Mr. R. was operated on. His condition improved markedly, and he went home to live a reasonably normal life.

Why did these two patients not receive adequate treatment for their conditions over a period of years?

The answer to this question throws an interesting light on a little appreciated problem in modern medical practice, one that has hardly been studied at all, at least as a problem of significance in our health care system.

It can be put into one word: competition.

As the well-to-do and middle classes have moved from the cities to the suburbs, so their physicians have followed them. In one suburban area we studied, the number of physicians doubled while the population in the same area increased by scarcely more than a third during the same period.

It is there, in the suburbs, that, from the private, traditional point of view of medical practice, the action is. The bulk of the physicians' patients now live here, and they are the patients he likes to treat because they are used to the old free-for-service principle of medical care and, most importantly, either have the money to pay for his services directly or are adequately covered by health insurance plans. The availability of both methods of payment is the foundation for such successful medical practices.

But imagine the competition! Put yourself into a young doctor's shoes. He needs to make a living, and he does it by treating sick people. In a fee-for-service situation, the more patients the doctor sees, and more frequently he sees them, the more money he makes. But the population available for medical treatment is not unlimited and there are other doctors only too eager to take on easy cases and well-paying chronic patients who form a source of long-term assured payments.

It is no wonder then that physicians can on occasion reach pretty far to keep their hands on their patients. We know of one case in which a patient transferred to another doctor in her neighborhood. She took a prescription from her new physician to be filled at the local pharmacy where she had always gone. The pharmacist refused to fill the order and called up the patient's former doctor to tell him that she was now consulting another man. Thus informed of his patient's "defection," the first physician phoned his ex-patient and requested that she appear forthwith in his office and explain herself. She refused.

In other words, physicians are in competition with each other for business, and their business is your body. The longer they can keep you coming to their door, the more it costs you—in time and money—and the more money they can make.

Thus Mrs. G.'s esophageal stricture remained improperly treated until finally good judgment prevailed on her part and her problem was correctly diagnosed and then properly treated. Likewise, Mr. R.'s circulatory condition, ultimately relieved by relatively simple cardiac surgery, remained undiagnosed, even at the cost of keeping the patient a permanent cripple.

It is impossible to prove, of course, that these patients were deliberately treated inadequately just to keep them on their doctors' books. The original diagnosis of scleroderma may have been due to simple ignorance, but although it is not rare, it can only be diagnosed definitively through careful laboratory tests and tissue pathology. If these had been properly done in Mrs. G.'s case, they would surely have ruled out scleroderma as her problem. But such a step could mean loss of face and possibly of a good source of revenue.

Shortness of breath does occur in chronic pulmonary disease but it is also a symptom of other things and in Mr. R.'s case these should have been considered at an early stage, instead of allowing years to elapse while the patient was labeled a pulmonary cripple, permanently disabled and removed from the mainstream of life.

The point is that these two patients—typical of many others—were treated for long periods of time without their symptoms being relieved. No good doctor should continue to treat patients under such conditions without obtaining a consultation with an independent authority on the particular medical problem involved. But considerations of personal ego and revenue loss prevailed.

However, in another and most important sense, the way that these two patients were treated—or ill-treated—was due to some extent to their own naiveté. No patient should be satisfied to be treated for years for a "chronic" condition without some outside review by a specialist. Every patient should insist on having an independent opinion on his problem. He is entitled to it. Indeed, in these days of rapid medical progress and the development of new therapies, only specialists are able to keep up with the most effective treatments in well-defined areas such as thoracic, cardiac, and vascular diseases.

The days when you could consider your doctor as some kind of father figure are gone—if they ever really existed. It is comforting and even occasionally therapeutically useful to have a pleasant, gray-haired, all-knowing physician who wisely nods his head at appropriate intervals, then gives you some pills. But don't mistake good bedside manners for good medicine.

When you need the best, get the best. When you don't, stay away from the entrepreneurs. They're a waste of time and money and, in the long run, of your health.

Perhaps nowhere is this point better exemplified than in the area of surgery. In 1970 there were over 75,000 surgeons actively practicing their specialty in this country, and the Parkinson principle applies: "Work expands with the increased availability of people to do it."

Because surgery is the largest single specialty in the medical profession, it is singled out as an example. But as far as you, the consumer, are concerned, the principle applies equally to all branches of medicine.

VI

The Unkindest Cut . . .

The main thrust of this book is that most medical services are vastly over-utilized; among such overused services, unnecessary surgery clearly holds the lead.

One good reason for this is the simple fact that there are more than twice as many surgeons as there are internists, the next largest medical specialty.

But this tells only part of the story, because only about seventy percent of the surgeons in the U.S. are in fact board-certified. In other words, almost one-third of the medically qualified individuals in this country who describe themselves as surgeons are not in fact qualified as surgeons by certification from the American Board of Surgery.

And there's more that makes your risk even greater. In a survey, published in the *Journal of Surgery* in March of 1972, of several community hospitals in the New York area, four surgeons reported that the surgeons who did the most work were the non-board-certified surgeons. Non-certified surgeons were performing three times more operations than were the semi-qualified surgeons and over 40 percent more than the fully board-certified surgeons.

There are over 15 million surgical procedures done in the United States every year. In 1965, the National Center for Health Statistics estimated the figure at 14 million. One half of all hospital admissions are for surgery of one kind or another.

Think very carefully before you let yourself or some member of your family become one of those 15 million patients! This is probably the most vitally important piece of advice in this whole book.

For some inexplicable reason, far too many normally sane individuals—who wouldn't hire a file clerk or a mail room boy without checking previous employers and amassing a reasonable amount of information on his past performance— seem perfectly willing to hop onto an operating table and let anyone with a license "to practice the healing arts" on his office wall (and a scalpel in his hand) open them up and rummage around in their interiors. The phenomenon has not gone unnoticed by many good surgeons themselves, but as a professional body they have done virtually nothing either to educate the patient so that he at least pauses and thinks before he lets a surgeon go to work on him, or to prevent the less scrupulous among their professional number from taking advantage of this human quirk.

So it is up to you, the potential patient, to be very skeptical about any recommendation for surgery and to refuse to be rushed into it, however terrified you may be or however much the surgeon tries to brainwash you about the dire results of delay.

All surgery carries a possible risk of death, disability, or complications, depending on the type of operation or the absolute need for it. (You can find out what the risk is for your particular procedure by consulting some of the sources of information listed at the end of this book.) For example, there are about 300 deaths a year associated with tonsillectomies and adenoidectomies. Considering the number of such operations—currently over one and a half million a year in the U.S.—this percentage is extremely low, well within what surgeons call "acceptable limits." But remember —if your own little boy or girl is one of the 300, then it's 100 percent. And to add salt to the wound, the tonsillectomy is today considered by most surgeons of questionable value in seventy percent of the cases, although it is the most common operation in a listing of fifty operations most frequently performed.

A few years ago, a California anesthesiologist, Dr. John Bunker, of Stanford University Medical School, made a comparative study of British and American surgical practices. He found that in the United States 7,400 operations were performed annually per 100,000 people. In Britain, there were only 3,770 operations per 100,000 of the population—nearly half the number. Dr. Bunker cautioned that direct comparisons, using these overall figures, were not feasible, but where the operations were broken down by procedures, comparisons could be made with confidence. The number of hysterectomies performed, for instance, was twice as high in the U.S. as in Britain. Similarly, Dr. Bunker found the rate for many other types of operations such as gall-bladder removal, hemorrhoid surgery, and tonsillectomy and adenoidectomy were two or more times greater in the U.S. than in England and Wales.

It could be argued that because Americans have twice as much surgery, in some instances, as the English does not mean that these operations are unjustified. Perhaps the U.S.

enjoys the benefits of desirable surgical procedures that are not done in Britain because there surgery is only performed when absolutely needed. But nobody has as yet bothered to find out if we would be worse off with less surgery. Where figures do exist on the real need for operations, surgeons have not bothered to take advantage of the information. At least that is Dr. Bunker's contention. In Britain, surgery is rarely performed at the request of the patient or his referring physician.

Part of the difference in surgical patterns between Britain and the U.S. reflects a difference in national character. The American surgeon is more aggressive than his British counterpart. His *modus operandi* is: "Don't stand there. Do something." Possibly he has greater expectations of what surgery can do for his patient. The British surgeon is more cautious, perhaps more realistic. Faced with a case and uncertain how to proceed, he ponders, or at least delays action —thus perhaps allowing nature the chance to cure.

These national characteristics are not confined to doctors. The American patient is quite as likely to be eager to have the surgeon "do something." But it is also significant that there are more surgeons available in the U.S. and the patient's insurance will pick up the hospital and surgical tab. Also, more medical school graduates enter the surgical field in America than in Britain because they know they can make more money at it than in any other specialty. This, however, has nothing to do with the actual defined need for number of surgeons or surgery.

It is significant that prepaid health plans such as the Kaiser Permanente Group use only six general surgeons per 100,000 people, while under the usual fee-for-service system in the country at large, there are thirteen surgeons per

100,000 people. The result is to force up the amount of surgery performed since, after all, these surgeons have to make a living. Indeed it is our belief that dollars are the over-riding consideration of most practicing surgeons in the community hospitals of this country. There is seldom any definite criterion establishing the genuine need for any operation.

What is badly needed today is the establishment of rigid criteria for judging the genuine need for surgery. And since surgeons themselves apply little self-discipline in establishing these rigid criteria, it is up to the patient to question thoroughly the need for any surgical procedure before letting you or someone in your family go under the knife. This may be hard, at the time, if for instance you are in excrutiating pain from a kidney stone. But you should insist on relief of pain first then wait and see if the stone won't pass before you let a urological surgeon start probing your plumbing system. The damage he can do with cystoscopes and catheters is sometimes difficult to repair or may even be irreparable. Consider the following case history.

An elderly lady went to her doctor complaining of pain in her back and belly. Feeling her abdomen, the physician thought he detected an aneurysm of the aorta—a ballooning out of the main vessel that carries the blood to the lower part of the body. (Sometimes, when the vessel wall is very fragile, an aneurysm will burst, just as a tire blows out.)

So the doctor promptly put the old lady in the hospital and told her an operation would be necessary "to repair the aneurysm." He did no tests or X-rays. He just informed her he had found a surgeon who would do the procedure.

As her nearest relative, the patient's son was informed. Aware of the seriousness of the proposed surgery, he promptly checked up on the suggested surgeon by looking his name up in the *Directory of Medical Specialists.* This is available in most large libraries. Your own doctor probably has one. Here there is a full description of every man's career, his qualifications and where he was trained. The son found no indications that this particular surgeon was qualified in vascular surgery so he decided that he did not want him to operate on his mother. Instead, he located another man, a specialist in the field, whose credentials were more reassuring.

He then went to his mother's doctor and asked him to have this specialist brought in for consultation. When this surgeon examined the old lady, he ordered an aortogram— an X-ray of the blood vessel. He found no evidence of any aneurysm. "The aorta was a little tortuous and the patient was tense, so this may have accounted for the original diagnosis of an aneurysm," he pronounced diplomatically. He also suggested that no surgery be done at that time.

This story shows us a number of ways we can protect ourselves from unnecessary surgery. First, the son checked on the qualifications of the suggested surgeon, through that helpful reference book, the *Directory of Medical Specialists.* Whatever kind of specialist your doctor refers you to, he should be checked by you for his qualifications. Do not assume that because a man describes himself as a surgeon that he is necessarily qualified to perform the proposed operation. For example, a gynecologist would be as unlikely to undertake a delicate ear operation as an ear, nose, and throat specialist would be to deliver a baby (except possibly in an acute emergency). Although it may be hard to believe, only about two-thirds of those who describe themselves as surgeons have actually been passed as qualified in this specialty by a board of examiners. These non-qualified individuals also do not belong to the American College of Surgeons, a group with stringent professional requirements. So it is well to check to make sure your surgeon has the letters F.A.C.S. (Fellow—American College of Surgeons) after his name.

To return to the case just discussed, not only should the surgeon have been qualified in surgery but he should also have been a specialist in blood-vessel surgery. As additional security, the patient's son could have assured himself that he was a member of one or other of the societies of vascular surgery. This would have indicated that he was not only qualified but more likely than not he was reasonably competent. This holds for other surgical specialities—urology, obstetrics, chest surgery, and so on.

Having decided against the surgeon his mother's doctor recommended (who was simply someone on the staff of the local hospital and therefore readily available), and having found a suitable individual to consult, the patient's son was right to ask his mother's doctor to bring in this man as a consultant on the case. If the doctor had refused, the son could have removed his mother from the hospital and taken her to the surgeon's office himself.

Although you cannot bring in a consultant on a case by yourself as long as another physician is in attendance, you do have the right to request your doctor to ask a consultant of your choice (not the one he uses!) and if he refuses, you have the right to remove yourself or your loved one from his care.

In other words, you have the right *not* to take your doctor's advice. You have the right to be operated upon by a surgeon of your own choosing, and you need not be forced to stay in any hospital against your will. However, it is a good idea to excercise these rights intelligently, as this young man did. This way, he had his mother's doctor on their side.

While discussing this problem of the relationship of private physicians to medical specialists, we should make mention of fee-splitting. This means the referring doctor gets a portion of the fee that the specialist charges you—a sort of tip for passing on a patient. Fee-splitting is unethical and is frowned upon by the American Medical Association and the American College of Surgeons. It is even illegal in some states. Nonetheless, it does go on, in other forms such as receiving assistant's fees and fees for unnecessary aftercare.

You can't find out for sure whether your doctor is taking a kickback like this from a surgeon he has recommended to you. But you can suspect as much if your bill is higher than it should be. You can check the going rate for any surgical procedure through your insurance agent or even another doctor. If your bill is fat, it may have put on weight through a kickback. Apart from the fact that it is illegal in many states, fee-splitting is not a practice that the best specialists have to engage in because they have plenty of cases sent to them without having to tip the referring physician. They can also afford to be more objective than the specialist who knows some professional friend of his is waiting eagerly for a percentage of whatever may be charged for surgery or other treatment.

Let us repeat here that it is imperative to have a frank discussion of costs before you agree to any procedure, medical or surgical.

If any surgeon or physician recommends an operation for you, make him explain why. Ask him for a frank estimate of the risks involved. Good physicians and surgeons will tell you, sometimes even before you ask, and you should respect the man who says honestly that he doesn't know, and refuses to promise you a modern miracle. If you have any remaining doubts, indeed, as a general rule, say you want an independent consultation with *someone not associated with the original specialist or the same hospital.*

The value of a consultant is that he doesn't have any ax to grind. Provided he is not going to do the surgery himself, he can afford to be objective. His contribution to your own peace of mind can be inestimable, worth far more than the fee you pay him. Also, because you'll only see him once, you can often ask him questions you might hesitate to put to your own physician, or surgeon.

A young woman, recently recovered from complicated disc surgery, told us she had been emotionally sustained through a grueling convalescence by the information she had received from an independent neurologist, a professor at a medical school, before she consented to the surgery— which, incidentally, she had been told was most urgent to avoid paralysis of both legs. Fortunately for her, she had worked in the medical field, so knew what to ask. Here are some of the questions she put to the consultant:

1. How "routine" is this procedure? (In her case, she was told the hospital handled at least seven such operations a week, which meant they were experienced in handling these cases. She was also told that her particular surgeon usually got good results and was considered an expert in this particular field.)

2. What exactly will be done? (In her case, she was shown a model of the back and had the whole procedure explained so that she understood the need for the operation.)

3. Besides the area that is being cut, what other organs can be affected? Will the operation leave any permanent problems and what are these likely to be?

What danger signals signpost future problems, if any?

4. How "typical" is this case? What is the average age for this kind of surgery and what is the expectancy of full recovery?

5. What kinds of medication will be involved? (Here she sensibly told the consultant the drugs she took routinely for other complaints and satisfied herself that these would not conflict with those she was likely to be given in the hospital. Like many people, she was allergic to certain antibiotics and on the Pill.)

6. How long is the recuperative period? How long a stay in hospital is involved and—vitally important—what arrangements must be made for domestic help after going home? Would she, for instance, be able to do her housework and cope with two small children? How long would it be before she could return to her job? (She was told she would have to lie mostly flat on her back for several months, and although she could stand and walk, she could not bend. Since she could not sit in a chair for any length of time during the first few months, she could not use a typewriter or sew or pick up her baby. She could also expect to be taking painkilling drugs for some time, so her ability to concentrate—whether on her work or on her domestic duties—would be curtailed.)

7. How long would it be before she could resume her sex life? ("Reasonably soon," she was told, "as long as there were no acrobatics.")

8. What psychological effects did this operation have? (The consultant warned her that post-operative depression was standard, not simply because of the pain but because the patient had to be extremely passive. Trying to fight against weakness only slowed down recovery. To an active, determined individual, this meant a considerable adjustment—but at least she was forewarned.)

9. How soon could she drive her car, travel, visit friends, or entertain?

10. Finally, she asked the consultant what would happen if she did not have the operation at all?

It is surprising how many members of the medical profession don't know the answer to this final question. Dr. Bunker relates how he himself had a torn cartilage in his knee joint. He asked the orthopedic surgeon whom he consulted what would happen if he were not operated on? The specialist replied, "We really don't know because we have not ever *not* operated." Many authorities feel that half the disc operations in community hospitals need not have been done.

But in obtaining this information, you must also bear in mind that in medicine nothing is ever absolutely certain. The kind of answer you get to a medical question cannot be exact. Even though we all have a head, a body, two legs, and two arms, we aren't really alike. Far from it, each one of us is unique in many highly specialized ways. The way one person responds to a drug, a test, or to surgery may be quite different from the response of another individual, even from the same family.

This chapter has tried to indicate ways that you can protect yourself from unnecessary surgery. Besides the steps you can take as an individual, there are approaches that could be taken by authorities—medical, governmental and regulatory. One suggestion is that health insurers should not pay for procedures performed by surgeons unqualified to do the surgery they bill for. Both medical associations and state licensing boards, as well as hospitals, could take steps to ensure that only fully qualified men be allowed to perform specialist work. But these steps, if ever they are taken, are for the future. (See Chapter XVI.) At the moment, the onus is on you, the patient.

But to show how sometimes over-enthusiastic surgery can backfire on the surgeon, there is a possibly apocryphal story told by an internationally known physician about an obstetrician and gynecologist who, because he lived in a small town out West where there was a doctor shortage, also had a lucrative pediatric practice. He performed so many expensive hysterectomies on the local female populace that his palatial home was referred to behind his back as "The House That Uteri Built." Unfortunately, he overreached himself. He did so many hysterectomies that the town's birth rate fell and the doctor began to run out of patients. In the end, he ran out of money too, and by that time he was too old to move and begin practicing somewhere else.

VII

What Price Your Doctor?

"Well, George," said Dr. X, greeting a colleague in the country club locker room the other day, "how are you beating the price freeze?"

"Easy," George replied, "I just see more patients each day. Don't need to cram a lot more in, one or two at the most does it and no one notices the difference."

This exchange is fictional, but the point is not. Until recently, doctors who wanted to increase their income over the 2.5 percent allowed by the Price Commission were advised by their professional business magazine, *Medical Economics,* to do just that—add more patients to the daily schedule. Another suggestion was to add more items to the patient's bill.

Doctors have the highest income of any professional group in the country, according to the U.S. Census Bureau. They are followed by bankers, dentists, professors of medicine and lawyers, in that order.

The median net income of all medical doctors, according to the office of research and statistics of the Social Security

Administration, is $40,550 per year. Median net income is income after business expenses have been deducted but before taxes have been paid. The figure is for 1969, the latest year for which figures are available.

But some medical specialists make more than others. In 1969, obstetricians and gynecologists headed the list. Their median net annual income was $43,770. General surgeons were runners-up with $42,960. Internists followed with $38,350; general practitioners with $35,140; and pediatricians with $34,430.

Medical Economics, which periodically surveys physicians' incomes along with other economic facts of the medical man's life, confirms this figure. It reports that the median income of doctors under 65 years of age who are in private practice is somewhat over $40,000 a year. This is a considerably higher average income than that of a lawyer, which the American Bar Association puts at an average of $28,000 annually.

There have been many attempts made to find out why doctors earn more than any other professional group. None have been completely satisfactory. In part, it is due to the old economic principle of supply and demand. When the demand is high and the supply short, then the price rises, as the classical economist Adam Smith pointed out some two hundred years ago.

For a number of years the American Medical Association sought, with some success, to restrict entry into the medical profession as a matter of policy. In 1910, there were 164 doctors per 100,000 persons in the United States. In 1963 the number was 124 per 100,000. This trend has been reversed slightly. In 1967, there were 130 physicians per 100,000 population, and the number will certainly increase in the coming years. Twenty new medical schools have opened and the number of medical graduates has increased. It is up by one-third in the last twenty years.

The government plans to increase the total number of physicians in the U.S. to nearly 440,000 by 1978. Most authorities estimate that the country needs at least 50,000 more doctors. But the irony of the situation is that nobody knows how many doctors we really need or will need in the future.

One factor that all agree upon is that it is not just a matter of the number of physicians, it is their distribution, both in terms of geography across the country and within the profession in terms of specialization. It won't do much good mustering an army of nearly half a million doctors if the majority of them continue to set up shop in the already "well-doctored" neighborhoods. Nor is it likely to be beneficial if the majority of the medical school graduates continue to become specialist surgeons, as they are doing today. Our problems will in fact be compounded, because, as we have seen, the more surgeons we have, the more surgery they will do— regardless of whether the wielding of those scalpels is actually necessary.

All of this is to warn the consumer that there's more to the problem of physicians' shortage than numbers. Now let us get back to the present situation and in particular the doctor's bill and his income.

A favorite reason cited by doctors as an explanation of their high income is that they have given long years to study and they have worked at low rates of pay as interns and residents. They are, they say, merely catching up with the rest of the population when they set themselves up in practice. The argument sounds good, but it doesn't hold water.

It is true that most physicians spend up to ten years or

more in college and post-graduate education before they begin to earn a living at anything like their potential. But this time is not much more than that spent by dentists and lawyers. Further, the net average individual lifetime earnings for the medical profession are over $700,000, almost $100,000 more than a lawyer's.

Further, physicians' incomes have climbed very steeply in recent years, at almost double the cost of living. Government economists report that doctors' incomes have gone up 58 percent in the past ten years while in the same period the consumer price index as a whole has risen only 31 percent. This is a faster increase than any other medical cost except hospital services—and, we will see if there is some justification for their increased charges.

The continuing trend towards specialization in medicine is a factor that has certainly contributed to the increase in the doctor's bill. A specialist will charge two or even three times the fee of a general practitioner. Today, four physicians in five are specialists. Forty years ago, according to a survey done by the U.S. Department of Commerce, only one physician in four was a specialist. Ten years ago, the profession was equally divided between specialists and general practitioners.

This is not to say that what we pay for doctors' services is exactly a negligible amount. In fact, we are today grossly overcharged for our doctor services compared with only a few years ago.

According to the Bureau of Labor Statistics, in the months following the enactment of Medicare and the beginning of benefits under the program, one-third of all physicians' charges rose by 20 percent. From an annual increase of 2 to 3 percent in 1964-65, the doctors' charges went up by

4.2 percent in 1966; 7.5 percent in 1967; and 6.1 percent in 1968. By comparison, all the items in the consumer price index were increasing in the same period by only between 2 and 3.5 percent per year.

The net result is that today doctors' charges are one-fifth to one-third higher than they should be. This amounts in medical care costs to consumers of hundreds of millions of dollars since 1965.

While considering the influence of the doctor's bill on the consumer, it must also be pointed out that it takes only about 20 percent of the health dollar. Hospitals—taking 40 percent—have the largest bite. The real effect of the doctor on your purse is not so much his own fee as the frequency and variety of the tests and procedures that he orders.

There is much emotional discussion among laymen about how much doctors earn, but it is often surprising how frequently the patient will pay the doctor's bill without query. It is important that you, as a patient, do not accept unnecessarily high charges by your doctor on the assumption that you are therefore receiving high quality care. While it is true that good quality goods usually cost more than poor quality, the relationship does not necessarily follow automatically. Don't let yourself be overcharged, then fool yourself that you are getting better service in consequence. Keep it in mind that doctors have a higher income than any other profession, and there is no need for you to make unnecessary contributions to keep your practitioner in the higher tax brackets to which he has become accustomed.

The rapid growth of third party health insurance plans that started with the Blue Cross plans for hospital services and expanded into Blue Shield for coverage of medical services and subsequently into health insurance plans underwritten by commercial insurance companies have all helped to escalate the doctors' earnings. To a considerable extent, such plans ensure that the physician will be paid for his services regardless of the current state of his patient's bank balance. It has been estimated that about half the doctor's income, today, comes from such health insurance payments.

At the national level, where governments have become involved in reimbursement for medical services, sliding scales have been used together with cost control methods to keep down the expense of medical and surgical services. For example, in Canada the national health insurance plans are run in conjunction with the provincial governments and provide a system of basic health care for all. The overall cost of these programs, not only in terms of actual cash but in terms of unnecessary care, has been considerably reduced through a sliding scale pay system.

In Newfoundland, for example, the system provides for a 90 percent payment of the doctor's bill by the national and provincial governments and a 10 percent contribution by the patient. But this only holds good for payments below a fixed amount—$4,500 a month for the general practitioner, $5,500 for the specialists and $6,500 for surgical specialists. Above that level, only 75 percent of the next thousand dollars is paid on only 50 percent of any amount beyond that. Similar scaled-down reductions in payment have been imposed in Ontario and Quebec. There is evidence that this system makes it unprofitable for physicians or surgeons to undertake unnecessary medical or surgical care.

However, the debate over the doctor's income and how much he charges really obscures the main problem. Anne Somers, the well-known medical economist from Princeton

University, notes that the real issue today is how the doctor's economic status might stand in the way of providing good health care to a broader section of the population.

There are some hopeful signs on the horizon. A quarter century or even a decade ago, many individuals went into the medical profession for the sole purpose of making money. It is these people who have swollen the ranks of the medical specialties, especially surgery—the highest money-maker of the lot.

Today, we see signs that medicine is becoming less attractive to the self-seeking, get-rich-quick individual. One factor is the increasing complexity of medicine which tends to discourage the fee-for-service entrepreneur. Another is the possibility of greater regulation. This is implied by the growth of federal involvement in the health industry—the government now pays almost one-third of the nation's total health bill—which makes some form of control over the health professional inevitable. There is also a very definite trend toward the eventual development of a universal federal health insurance plan of one type or another with all that this implies in restrictions on both patients seeking services and physicians and other health professionals providing them.

This is only a clinical impression, for there are little hard data to support this view. The younger generation seems more idealistic than their parents, and many of today's medical students seem to be more interested in medicine than in money. They are more concerned with the economic plight of patients. It is possible that the next generation of physicians may be more likely to put these patients before their pocketbooks and thus restore some badly needed self-respect to a profession which has recently, if sometimes unfairly,

been accused of grasping self-interest with little feeling for
their patients.

VIII

The Hasty Heart Attack

James T. is a stout, pleasant, ruddy-faced man of 46, with an attractive wife and two children. He is an electronics engineer in the $20-30,000 a year income bracket. Last year he had a sudden pain in his chest. He phoned his family physician, Dr. R., who told him to go at once to the local hospital, where arrangements would be made to admit him immediately to their coronary care unit with a diagnosis of myocardial infarction—a possible heart attack.

After three days of intensive care, Mr. T. felt better, and in two weeks he was home with no definite EKG or laboratory evidence of any myocardial infarction—but with strong advice from his doctor to take it easy. The implication made was that Mr. T. had probably had a mild heart attack. No one told him otherwise, and he accepted this suggested diagnosis without question and felt duly grateful to the doctor for such prompt care, possibly saving his life. For months after, he went to his doctor for a weekly checkup, with the taking of blood specimens and an electrocardiogram. Each visit, although results were negative, reinforced his own belief that he had had a heart attack and that his doctor was a fine, thorough physician because "he pulled me through."

But did Mr. T. really have a heart attack? There was no biochemical or electrocardiographic evidence that his heart muscle had ever been damaged.

To be sure, he was overweight and his blood cholesterol level was somewhat high for his age. And Mr. T. certainly did experience that pain in his chest. But, at the time, according to the case records, his blood pressure was not abnormally high, and X-rays of his heart found it to be normal. Thus Mr. T. was the victim of a non-disease for which he received extensive management and tests. Following these, and intensive care, he was left physically and emotionally crippled. Not so incidentally, he also served to push up the cost of his own and the national medical care by being treated in the coronary care unit and by repeated laboratory tests.

Mr. T., in other words, had been enslaved by modern medical practice. What is worse, he didn't realize it. To him, it was the miracles of today's care that saved his life.

It seems incredible, when physicians are said to be in such short supply, and so overworked, and when so many people are really ill and need a doctor's services, that this could happen. But it did.

It happened because Mr. T. had money to pay for medical care, so medical care was standing by, only too ready to take care of him—for a fee, of course. Mr. T.'s doctor was richer by some $300 to $500 as a result of the "episode," and he continued to be paid for the subsequent checkups. Mr. T.'s health insurance plan footed these bills. The coronary care unit at the local hospital collected another $600 and about $300-500 went in laboratory tests and electrocardiograms.

Mr. T. wasn't personally impoverished. His company health plan paid all but $100.

The real tragedy that Mr. T.'s case represents is not the medical overcare or the role he played in forcing up medical care costs, but that the whole incident was avoidable. If Mr. T. had been sharper about purchasing his medical services and checking up on them as he bought them—in other words, if he had had a better doctor and a second, independent, opinion—he might not have had the experience.

Mr. T. had partially brought it upon himself. He had let himself be conditioned by the climate of today's public opinion to expect that a sudden pain in the chest might be a heart attack. He had also been led to believe that being hooked up to an electronic monitoring device represented the best and most modern medical care.

His doctor backs up this point of view. "Isn't it better to be in the coronary care unit, just in case it *might* be a heart attack?" he argues. "Then if some abnormality does develop, everything is at hand to save the patient's life?" This is the rationale. It seems sensible on its face. But is it?

What Mr. T.'s doctor either didn't know or didn't tell his patient was that *half the people admitted to a coronary care unit in the average community hospital turn out to have no evidence of a heart attack* when serial electrocardiograms and enzyme studies are done. Enzyme analyses will show the presence of tissue damage occurring after a heart attack and these, coupled with abnormalities in the electrocardiogram, confirm a diagnosis of a myocardial infarction.

Moreover, even if he actually had a heart attack, there was no good reason why Mr. T. should have been sent straight to the coronary care unit. Only about 10 to 20 percent of the patients with heart attacks admitted to community hospitals ty hospitals need monitoring because of irregularity of cardiac rhythm. These units cost up to $200 a day, per patient, depending on the hospital, and up goes the medical bill accordingly.

Incidentally, the type of care that is given today's cardiac patient is cited by some physicians as the reason why costs of medical care are rising. Their argument runs something like this. Twenty years ago, a heart attack led to a brief hospital stay and death—assuming the patient even got to a hospital. If a man is returned to a useful productive life by the aid of modern drugs and devices instead of being buried in his grave, then he continues to contribute to the total productivity of society by earning a living and paying his taxes. All this would have been lost if he had died. Thus the true cost of the modern equipment in a hospital's coronary care unit is actually a saving—provided it is used properly.

This is the whole point of our criticism. If half the heart attacks are not really heart attacks at all, then this is a reflection on the incompetence of the medical profession in failing to diagnose the condition properly. We're not saying that all possible heart attacks can be diagnosed with 100 percent accuracy, but a 50 percent failure in diagnosis is hardly tolerable and is certainly wasteful of resources.

Mr. T.'s doctor, of course, faced a problem that has recently loomed very large in medicine. He was afraid that if he didn't do *everything,* he could be sued for malpractice, in the event Mr. T. developed an abnormal rhythm in the heart beat and possibly died. The family could say the doctor had not taken the proper steps to prevent this.

But if that doctor had taken the time to practice a little medicine, if he had examined his patient instead of depositing him, unseen, straight into the hospital's coronary care unit, he might have saved Mr. T. a lot of time, worry, and unnecessary expense. If, after examining his patient, the doctor had not felt Mr. T. needed intensive coronary care, he could have explained why and so blunted any threat of legal action, later on.

A goodly number of physicians have let the law dictate the way they practice medicine. Any man can be sued. That this happens is not necessarily a reflection on the ability or lack of it on the part of the physician. Beware the physician whose medical judgments are made in the light of what the courts may decide is good medical practice.

The chest pain seemed an emergency to Mr. T., and he and his wife were, naturally, scared. So, possibly, was the doctor. But once the emergency was over and he was safely in the hospital, Mr. T. should have been examined by a cardiologist. If his own doctor did not suggest such a specialist, Mr. or Mrs. T. should have found one, independently, and learned the true state of his health.

For a physician to try to find out what is wrong and then to tell the patient what is being done—or not done—and why, takes time. Many physicians won't take this time. They have taken advantage of modern technology and used it as a substitute for good medical practice. To be sure, time is the one thing a physician never has enough of. Under the present fee-for-service system of medical practice, he must see a certain number of patients in a day to keep ahead of his own running expenses.

Most doctors strenuously deny it, but they are just as surely on an assembly line as any factory worker. They simply have a little more flexibility. A doctor can buy time from Patient X who can safely be put off until next week (with a few pills), to spend more time with Patient Y who needs immediate treatment. But this doesn't alter the principle that to earn enough money to satisfy his own needs, a doctor must see a minimum number of patients in a day or charge more for those he does see.

This is one reason why so many medical men shrug off questions by their patients. One doctor has described his fellow professionals as the greatest egomaniacs in the world. They can't believe anyone else can be as smart as they are. "You wouldn't understand." "It's too complicated." "Now, Doctor knows best." "We're told we should always give these tests. Everyone should have them, regularly." The catch phrases are echoed every day by doctors.

Don't accept these non-answers to your legitimate questions. The idea that a layman can't understand something about medicine—especially as it concerns himself—is arrant nonsense.

With some help from an intelligent and patient doctor, and by using a little commonsense and understanding, anyone can learn something about what his doctor is doing and why he is doing it. Indeed, the whole point of this book is that since the doctor may not take the trouble to inform the patient fully, that patient had better learn something about medicine himself, or at least get some independent, outside professional consultation. If he doesn't, he's letting himself in for trouble.

It was this lack of knowledge, failure to inform himself, and perhaps being overly impressed with some of the tools of another man's trade that kept Mr. T. in trouble. He might still be going around thinking of himself as "a cardiac cripple" if he had not lost his job nine months after his "attack."

At his age, and with his health record (which company insurance carriers didn't like), he found it difficult to find any employment, until he was lucky enough to find a company that needed his particular kind of expertise. This organization took the trouble to check his health record with an independent consultant, a cardiologist. This expert, after studying the hospital files, discovered that the "heart attack" had probably been no more than a spasm of the coronary arteries or a bout of indigestion.

Mr. T. was once more healthy and happy.

IX

Community Hospitals

The medical profession has been called a priesthood. If you choose to look at it this way, then the hospital is the physicians' temple, for good medicine, today, is inseparable from the hospital.

In nine cases out of ten, if you are really sick, the hospital is the only place where your doctor can give you adequate treatment, because it has diagnostic laboratories, well-equipped operating rooms, and intensive care units all under one roof.

It wasn't always this way. Before the turn of the century, hospitals were largely custodial institutions for people who were too sick to be nursed to health at home, or who had to be isolated because of infectious diseases. Treatment was not likely to cure. What was given was of necessity just supportive, because there was actually very little that a hospital or doctor could then do except let nature take its course. If you had undergone surgery, you stood an 80 to 90 percent chance of dying from wound infection—assuming you survived the shock of the operation in the first place. If you were lucky enough not to pick up another disease or infection while you were in the hospital, you recovered.

Then, about fifty years ago, came the great scientific advances in therapeutic medicine and surgery—in particular, the control of infection and the development of anesthesia. Hospitals began to take on their modern look. They became places for the definitive treatment—and cure—of disease. This process is still going on. Hospitals are less and less places for just nursing along the sick, and more and more places where disease is actively treated.

There are four main types of hospitals in this country. One is the city or municipal hospital. This institution is the descendant of the old-fashioned charity hospital of the nineteenth century—a charitable institution for the poor and dispossessed.

Second, there is the large medical center. Like the city hospital, it is usually, although not always, in the downtown section of a large metropolitan district. Today, it is also likely to be closely affiliated with a medical school or participating in a teaching program. The professional staff have teaching appointments at the medical school. The standard of care is high, because of close supervision by the medical educators.

The third variety is the community hospital. We will be discussing these institutions in some detail later, so suffice to say here that they are supposed to be non-profit and tax-free, and they are usually run by a professional hospital administrator and staff responsible to a board of trustees composed of prominent local business and professional men, who serve without pay.

The fourth type of hospital is the profit-making institution or proprietary hospital. In general, the quality of medical care in such places is not as good as in other types of hospitals. But, if you have plenty of money, and are not very ill, such a hospital can serve you adequately. As a matter of guidance, however, stay out of a proprietary hospital if you face major surgery or have a serious medical disorder.

Recently there has been a rapid growth of the profit-making hospitals and nursing homes. Anne Somers, an authority on health care organization, notes that there are now a hundred corporations engaged in the business of providing institutional health services. Some of these places have shown a capacity to operate at significantly lower costs than community or other large hospitals. This is probably because they do not provide unduly complicated medical services or therapy calling for expensive equipment that is only used occasionally.

Generally speaking, the more serious your illness or contemplated surgery, the better off you will be in a major medical center than in a smaller community hospital, because the process of active disease treatment is further advanced in a large, well-supervised institution. You may not be as comfortable, or have color TV in your room, but, as a sick person, you stand a better chance of getting out alive and well.

However, something has happened since the end of World War II that makes it more likely you will be treated in a community hospital today than in a major medical center.

Since the late 1940s, there has been a steady movement of population to the suburbs. To serve this population, and aided by federal subsidies such as the Hill-Burton Act and funds raised locally, community hospitals have expanded beyond all recognition. They now deliver a substantial portion of the primary medical and surgical care to the middle and upper-middle classes who live in these suburban communities.

With the decline of the cities as residential areas for the well-to-do, the large urban medical center with its teaching staff and research programs has decreased its services to the paying patient.

This might not have potentially serious consequences to you as a patient if it were not for the extremely rapid growth of modern therapeutic techniques in medicine and surgery. The community hospital which has grown up to accommodate the enlarged suburban population, has frequently installed new devices and gadgets. But all too often, it has not paralleled this growth, intellectually. In other words, it does not necessarily have the well-qualified and self-disciplined staff and the institutional motivation to provide the kind of care that is possible in the context of today's medical discoveries.

Indeed, with its heart-lung machines, million-volt radiation equipment, intensive care units, and the host of therapeutic weapons of immense power and sophistication at its disposal, the community hospital is in something of the position of the small boy who, given a physics set for Christmas, has just constructed an atom bomb.

This point was clearly demonstrated in two recent studies. One involved the use of open-heart surgery units, the other X-ray equipment. In *The Annals of Thoracic Surgery,* Dr. J. Gordon Scannel of Harvard Medical School and his associates found that of 62 responses to a questionnaire they sent to 87 surgical centers in the U.S. inquiring about the use of open-heart surgery units, only 25 centers met what they regarded as the minimal requirements for efficient open-heart surgery—the practical experience of undertaking four to six such operations every week. Anything less is not

only unproductive but, what is worse, the surgeons operating
a unit cannot maintain sufficient skill and expertise. In one
community hospital near Boston, only two open-heart operations were performed in one year—and one of the patients
died on the operating table.

Dr. Scannell also concluded that only 25 open-heart surgery units were really necessary to serve the entire United
States. Yet open-heart surgery units continue to be installed
in smaller hospitals where there is not enough skilled support, partly because of insufficient use of the unit. Moreover,
their cost ultimately appears on the patient's total medical
bill—and pushes it up.

In the study on X-ray equipment use, reported in the
New England Journal of Medicine, there were wide varia-
tions in cost and effectiveness of radiation therapy among 67
hospitals surveyed in Massachusetts, New Hampshire, and
Rhode Island. Of the 67 hospitals surveyed, only 15 provided
any significant number of radiation therapy treatments. One
hospital had given no therapy at all in over a year, while
another treated only 25 patients annually.

In the hospitals that did not treat many patients, most of
the treatments were for benign conditions, less than one-
third were receiving radiation for cancer.

On the other hand, while the hospitals with a larger load
of patients receiving radiotherapy treated malignant conditions—as many as 95 percent of the patients treated at four
university-associated hospitals were being treated for cancer
—from one-quarter to one-third were being treated for recur-
rent disease.

This, points out Dr. B. S. Bloom of Harvard Medical
School, author of the study, is striking. It means "that the
major centers are treating patients with palliative therapy

when they should have been providing the primary treatment, while the smaller hospitals were giving primary treatment when they should have been administering palliation."

It has already been noted by others that the survival rates in patients given radiation for cervical cancer are better where the hospital treats large numbers of patients than in hospitals treating few such cases with radiotherapy. This has been attributed to better physical facilities and greater experience on the part of the staff.

Dr. Bloom and his colleagues concluded that five radiation centers would be sufficient to treat all the patients needing radiotherapy in the three states they surveyed—rather than the sixty-seven units currently in operation. The result would certainly be a considerable saving in X-ray facilities and skilled personnel.

The whole question of how hospitals are equipped and staffed is of such paramount importance to you in protecting yourself against poor medicine, that we are going to spend the rest of this and the next few chapters discussing the growth and development of a hospital serving a typical suburban community. We hope this will help you to recognize and evaluate both the strengths and the weaknesses of your own local community hospital.

The Blackstone Community Hospital, as we shall call it, serves a population that, in the three years from 1968 to 1971, has grown by 30 percent. This population now stands at about 100,000. In 1968, the area was served by one hospital of 250 beds. Since then, this hospital has added another 150 beds, and a new 320-bed wing has been built.

So the community now has 700 beds available—more than twice the number of hospital beds for an increase of just under one-third of the population.

In 1968, there were 75 practicing physicians in the area. Today there are 200. This is a ratio of one doctor for every 500 people—one of the highest in the country. The area served by the Blackstone Community Hospital is one of the fastest-growing bedroom communities in the U.S.A. and is a well-doctored district. Indeed, it might be considered "over-doctored" and this, as we will see, can be hazardous to a patient's health.

Unfortunately, most of this increase in medical personnel is reflected in the various specialties. Only one doctor in five is a general practitioner, and only one new man has been added to this field in the three years under discussion. On the other hand, the number of internists rose from five to fifteen, and the number of general surgeons from six to fifteen, so these two specialties now lead the field. The increases in other medical and surgical specialties are as follows: chest surgeons from one to six; orthopedic surgeons from three to nine; urologists from two to seven; ear, nose and throat specialists from two to six; ophthalmic surgeons from two to six; obstetricians from three to eight; radiologists from two to nine; pathologists from two to four; and anesthesiologists from three to seven.

All these specialists use the Blackstone Community Hospital and the heart of the health care delivery problem is in the organization of the hospital's staff.

Until modern times, hospitals were the private reserve of the medical profession where the doctors roamed more or less unhindred and unquestioned by administrators or boards of trustees. What the doctor wanted, the doctor got. When "Doctor" ordered, the staff jumped to obey. The administrator and his staff only handled the bills. The trustees were there to give the hospital the proper aura of public service—

since, after all, it was a tax-free institution. Neither of these last two groups had much influence on the medical men.

Today, this picture is changing. In many hospitals, particularly the bigger ones, public concern over rising costs, the closer association of medical schools with hospitals, the matter of legal responsibility for the actual care that goes on in a hospital, and not least, the public's concern over the quality and availability of the medical care provided there have all combined to force changes on the hospital.

But these changes have not as yet been felt at Blackstone. And this is the problem for its patients.

Medicine, by tradition in the United States, is organized in a hierarchical system. In most hospitals there are usually two senior chiefs—the chief of medicine and the chief of surgery. Under them are the chiefs of departments such as obstetrics and gynecology (which is under surgery) and the department of internal medicine (which falls within the chief of medicine's responsibility). There are often other important appointments such as the director of medical education and a similar position in surgery.

The rest of the medical staff is composed of attending physicians and surgeons, and frequently these days a number of residents, younger doctors, recently graduated and in training for some specialty.

When such a system is run by people of high ideals and standards, it works well. It ensures stability, yet can absorb change. It works for the benefit of the patient, who gets the benefit of the newest forms of therapy but is protected by the chain of authority from being exposed to untried or unproven methods of treatment.

As can be appreciated, the hierarchical system depends heavily upon the senior men for its effectiveness. If they encourage high quality, the hospital will be efficient and provide good care. But if the chiefs are not censorious of poor medical practice, the foundations are laid for tragedy to the patients.

It is of the essence in the hierarchical system that the authority is vested in the senior men. They control the hospital privileges of the doctors who practice in the area and decide what they can do within the hospital and what they can't.

This may sound efficient, but the system is only as good as the men who run it. The medical staff at Blackstone is composed of 80 percent specialists and 20 percent general practitioners. This is about the national average. But there are gaps in the specialties. Less than half of the internists, for example, are board certified. There is, for example, no cardiologist on the staff. Yet in a single year, 1970, over 7,000 electrocardiograms had been taken. A cardiologist is an expert who, among other things relating to the heart, is trained in reading the signs of heart disease as revealed by the heart wave machines, the electrocardiogram (EKG).

So why no cardiologist at the Blackstone Hospital? The explanation is revealing. The hospital, in 1970, collected $10 for each electrocardiogram, all read by the chief of the medical department who was reimbursed at the rate of $5 apiece. So, in this one year, he had collected approximately $35,000 for reading EKGs. Naturally he resisted appointing a cardiologist to the staff.

The department of surgery revealed the same pattern: the chief of general surgery frequently performed operations for which he was not trained or qualified, such as major blood vessel and chest surgery. Needless to say, the consequences were often disastrous for the patient, although lucrative to this particular surgeon. Since the chiefs themselves are guilty of such gross excesses, they can hardly be expected to control those under them adequately. Therefore, they allow other semi-qualified specialists to engage in similar practices.

How widespread across America is this kind of bad medical practice? It took three years to assemble the data on Blackstone Hospital, and the investigation took professional medical skill to evaluate the activities of the staff and also inside observation of how the hospital was actually organized.

There are many set-ups like Blackstone across the country. And because the population continues to move to the suburbs, such hospitals will continue to play a major role in providing medical and surgical service, despite the fact that the normal constraints on medical practice all too often do not work in these hospitals as they do in large medical centers. In teaching hospitals or large urban institutions no general surgeon, short of a dire emergency, would be permitted to operate on a patient with a serious blood vessel disorder such as an aneurysm. If he did, he would have to do so under the supervision of a good specialist in this field. The same goes for the inadequately qualified physician who treats seriously ill heart patients or, indeed, any other acute specialized problem. In the major medical centers, not only must the man who does the job be qualified to do it, but what he does will be carefully reviewed afterwards by a group of his professional peers.

But in the smaller institutions, where the chiefs are less self-disciplined, the staff becomes lax and the patient suffers. Such laxity, as we shall see, also plays an important part in forcing up health care costs through excessive and often unnecessary treatments, surgery, and other services.

Here is a typical case history that indicates not only the

kind of thing that can happen but also what you, as a patient, can do about it.

Mrs. Nancy G. found she needed two wisdom teeth extracted. Her dentist advised her to go into the Blackstone Hospital for the extraction because, he pointed out to her, if he did it in his office, she would have to pay for the minor surgery herself. But if she was hospitalized the cost would be covered by the health insurance plan provided by her husband's office.

Mrs. G. liked the idea because she was interested in the local Blackstone Hospital. Young, energetic, and community-minded, she knew the chief of surgery who had, indeed, encouraged her to raise a considerable sum of money toward new positive-pressure breathing equipment. This she had done through various women's clubs that she belonged to. So, to a small extent, she felt it was "her" hospital, though she had never, previously, been inside its doors, as a patient.

She was a little dismayed to find she had to check in the afternoon before she had her two teeth out, since this meant lining up a babysitter to stay with the children until her husband got home from work. She was told, however, that hospital regulations required patients be admitted the day prior to surgery. So she rationalized that she could rest up, relax with a book, or watch color television.

This, however, was not the way it was. She had scarcely had time to unpack her overnight bag before a succession of efficient-looking young people in white started barging into her room and submitting her to all kinds of tests. They drew two samples of her blood for analysis, took a urine specimen, and hooked her onto a large, portable machine for an electrocardiogram.

"Do you use the new breathing machine a lot?" Mrs. G.

asked the young woman who gave her this test.

"Yes—we do!" she replied, "and it's a curious thing. Before we had that machine, we had very few calls for it. But now we seem to be using it all the time. I guess," she added, packing up her machine, "when you have the equipment available, you find a use for it."

(This is true. At Duke University Medical Center, a few years back, one inhalation therapist gave positive pressure treatment to an average of eight patients daily. Since they've had extra machines, three therapists give the treatment to 95 patients every day.)

"And why do I have to have a chest X-ray?" Mrs. G. asked the next visitor. "I'm only having a couple of wisdom teeth out."

"Everyone who comes into this hospital has to have certain tests. They're regulation," she was told.

On her way to the radiology laboratory, she met a woman she knew in the hall. This patient was there for the removal of a small wart on her foot, and eager to talk about it.

"There's an empty bed in my room," she said. "Why don't you move in with me, and we can visit?"

But that was frowned upon by the administration. "You must be in a private room," Mrs. G. was told. "There could be a danger of infection, after your extraction. You can go and see your friend this evening."

Next morning, she had the two wisdom teeth out, and as she was being wheeled back to her room, she asked the attendant: "How soon can I check out? My husband's staying off work so he can drive me home, but he does want to go into the office later on."

"You can't leave until one of the doctors has seen you.

But someone will be along shortly."

When the doctor did appear, he was carrying a file with the results of her tests. "I'm afraid I've got some rather bad news for you," he told her. "Your blood specimen shows a proliferation of white cells."

White cells . . . leukemia . . . Mrs. G.'s heart missed a beat. "Wh—what does that mean?"

"Well," the doctor shrugged his shoulders, "perhaps nothing at all—possibly a temporary situation caused by the infected teeth. Or perhaps," he paused, "a more serious condition. You would be well advised to have some more tests. Who is your doctor?"

"I don't have a doctor. I go to a gynecologist, and of course we have a pediatrician for the kids, but . . . my husband and I are just never sick. . . ." She sat up in bed. "Look, my husband's waiting for me to call, to come by and pick me up. Surely I don't need any more tests right now?"

"Well . . . you'd have to come here again but," he smiled reassuringly, "you can go home today. Talk it over with your husband. And if you need any advice, I'm Dr. Michael R., and my office number is in the telephone book."

"You take private patients?"

"Yes indeed. . . ."

But Mrs. G. never called Dr. R. As an intelligent woman, she was beginning to have her reservations about Blackstone Hospital. "If they hadn't insisted on these tests they'd never have known there was anything wrong," she told her husband, "and I feel fine!"

"If it's anything serious, honey, you must have the best," he replied. "I'll ask our company medical department who the top blood specialists are at the city university center."

So, some weeks later, Mrs. G. went into town and saw

another doctor, who gave her another blood test. "I don't like to trust other people's results," he explained. "I'm afraid it costs the patient a little more—but it's a double check on the condition."

There was nothing abnormal about Mrs. G.'s blood.

"That increase in white cells could have been due to the infected teeth," the specialist said. "At any rate, it was a temporary situation." He smiled. "That hospital might even have mixed up your blood sample with someone else's. . . . We'll never know. But you can rest assured—there's nothing wrong with you."

There are several lessons to be learned from Mrs. G.'s experience. In the first place, she had no business going into a hospital for a procedure that could have been done in her dentist's office.

Secondly, by docilely going there she put herself into the clutches of an institutionalized system which operates regardless of circumstances. Had she phoned the admission office before she went there, she would have learned about all the tests and she might have revised her plans.

Thirdly, through receiving tests that had little or no relationship to her reason for being in the hospital, she—through her health insurance plan—was being used to amortize laboratory facilities that should only have been used in cases of real disease.

Finally, it was only because she herself questioned the system—and went outside of it for verification—that she escaped more testing and possibly even treatment for a disease she never had.

X

Who Really Runs the Hospitals

Nothing in this day of inflation has risen faster than hospital costs. The average expense per patient per day in a community hospital has risen by 38 percent from 1965 to 1968—in plain figures, from about $56 to $76 a day. And this is only what it costs the hospital. Needless to say, this increase is reflected in the patient's bill. At Blackstone, in the early 1970s, the charges range between $75 and $85 a day. Intensive care costs $150 to $200 a day. In 1968, the comparable figures were $45 for ordinary care and $100 for intensive care per day.

Future costs are expected to go even higher. Former American Hospital Association President, Mark Berke, and a former Assistant Secretary for Health at the Department of Health, Education, and Welfare, Dr. Philip Lee, have estimated that by the end of this decade, costs will average $100 a day in major urban hospitals, $600 in medium-sized community establishments like Blackstone, and $400 in rural areas. In short, hospital costs are out of control and nobody knows what to do about it.

91

No single item of medical care takes as large a slice out of the health dollar as the hospital. Although all costs of medical care have gone up in recent years, hospital costs have increased by the greatest amount—fivefold.

The reasons for this extraordinary increase in hospital costs have never been fully or even adequately analyzed. However, there are a number of good explanations, apart from inflation, as to why they have risen so steeply.

Salaries contribute the largest single factor. In 1967, the federal minimum wage law was applied to hospital staffs. This has doubled, in some cases tripled, the hospital's payroll expenditure, even when they employ the same number of people.

In recent years, as hospitals have been forced to improve working conditions for their staffs, they have had to employ more people. Where once they could get away with two people for a 24-hour shift, they now have to employ three. In community hospitals, between 1963 and 1968, the number of employees went up 13 percent.

More skilled technical help is needed today because of the enormous growth in medical technology over the past twenty years. For example, open heart surgery, as a practical therapeutic procedure, is less than twenty years old. Quite apart from the capital investment involved in purchasing the necessary equipment, such as heart-lung machines, for such surgery, highly trained technical help is required to man it.

The cost of the house staff is another reason for increases in hospital costs. Dr. John Knowles, until recently general director of the Massachusetts General Hospital, has said that when he was an intern there in 1951 his annual salary was $300. Today the beginning intern is paid $8,000 a year.

But even when all these factors and many others are taken

into account, the voluntary community hospital is plagued with a diffuse managerial structure which, as the health care authority Anne Somers points out, prevents the hospital "from fully employing the managerial controls essential to balance the new technologies and higher personnel earnings with increased productivity."

It has been fashionable to call medicine a cottage industry in a technological age. Nowhere is this more evident than in the voluntary community hospital. We hinted at the problem in the last chapter when we described the central position occupied by the medical staff.

In the absence of government or marketplace controls, a hospital administrator responds to other pressures. Even when he is determined to keep his hospital on a businesslike footing and in step with reality, the administrator is all too often defeated by the dual lines of authority and the vulnerability to persuasion by the medical staff or the hospital's board of trustees.

Hospitals must attract and keep a qualified medical staff, and this puts pressure on them to install new devices and the latest equipment—all in the name of improved services. The community in its turn is often led to regard the purchase of some brand-new diagnostic or therapeutic device as a mark of progress.

These forces exert pressure on the hospital administrator to demand that the hospital outfit itself with these trappings of prestige and status, regardless of whether the community needs such devices, and sometimes even when there is no properly qualified individual available locally to operate them. At Blackstone Hospital, for example, there are only five board-certified internists and not one of these individuals is a professionally trained cardiologist. Yet, regardless of this, fifteen attend patients in the intensive care unit.

In 1969, a group of American physicians under the chairmanship of Dr. Lester Breslow, head of the department of preventive medicine at the University of California, Los Angeles, undertook to look into American health services from the point of view of the cónsumer. Their report, which appeared in 1971, is required reading for anyone interested, as you are, in the problems of how health care systems should serve the patient.

One of the subjects this report takes up is just this problem of providing prestigious services even when the need is being met elsewhere in the community. Here, in part, is what it says:

"The buyer of the new medical technology does not generally have the specialized knowledge or the time to evaluate the product or to figure out how much it should cost him. With literally hundreds of companies competing for a share of the market for such devices as electrocardiographs, defibrillators and patient monitors, the average hospital administrator or the average physician is in no position to determine whether a particular feature of one model, which adds several thousand dollars to the cost, is really important or whether it is merely the medical electronics equivalent of a chromium tail fin.

"Second there is no reason to think that the hospitals are particularly concerned about the cost of the devices they buy. In the final analysis the hospitals don't pay the bill anyhow. The consumer pays, directly or through a third party, Blue Cross, Medicare, etc. The insurers pay the hospitals whatever the hospital claims was its actual cost of providing service. If the hospital buys and operates a computer, or an intensive care unit, the cost of providing a day's services rises. Automatically, the rate at which Blue Cross, Medicare and Medicaid reimburse the hospitals also rises.

"But even more seriously, as the report goes on to point out, "the greatest costs may be to the general community. For the money, manpower and physical resources directed to these prestigious frills might otherwise have provided needed health care. Indeed, even where expensive sophisticated equipment (or services) is not a frill, its purchase represents a setting of priorities, an establishing of values by which the entire community must live."

It is one of the fascinating, and to the conscientious hospital administrator, frustrating aspects of the present hospital system, that the non-profit, community hospital is overseen by a board of trustees, usually successful businessmen in the community, who wouldn't for a moment countenance the same practices of administration in their own businesses. Indeed, the trustees are often largely to blame for allowing hospitals to engage in loosely controlled purchasing and other procedures. New equipment can add to overall rising costs because it allows for more and more diagnostic and therapeutic procedures—which must be paid for by the patient, to justify its purchase.

The trustees, being non-medical men and women, are easily convinced that whenever a chief of medical services says he needs a new piece of equipment, the request is reasonable. They do not stop to consider how often it may be utilized—or that there may be such a device standing idle at some other, nearby hospital. So they readily agree to fresh purchases. After all, they argue, don't we want to provide the best possible care in our own hospital?

Another aspect inherent in the hospital trustee system is

that those who give their time to the voluntary hospital in
their community by serving as trustees are generally successful businessmen, lawyers and bankers, executives, members
of the accounting professions, and spokesmen for medicine
and hospitals. Dr. Theodore Goldberg of Wayne State University School of Medicine in Detroit and Ronald Hemmel-
gram, director of planning and research for the Community
Health Association, found in a review that half of hospital
board memberships were made up of businessmen, executives,
managerial personnel, small business owners, contractors,
realtors, investors, manufacturers and insurance represen-
tatives. About 13 percent of hospital trustees were drawn
from non-health professionals, lawyers for the most part.
Another 13 percent was made up of health professionals such
as dentists, optometrists, nurses and pharmacists, and the
remainder included religious professionals like ministers
and nuns. The patient, as a consumer of health care, was
little represented, if at all, the Wayne State study found.

Because they are shrewd businessmen themselves, many of
these trustees tended to confuse, if not actually equate, financial success with professional excellence. Physicians
make a lot of money. So it follows, in the thinking of the
business community, the wealthy doctor must also be a good
doctor and know what he's about, because he is successful.

It is also highly likely that the chiefs of services at the hospital are the medical advisors of the members of the Board
of Trustees. If so, this gives the medical man a chance to exercise a unique kind of pressure. Once a man gets his clothes
off and is in the examining room, it can be hard to resist a
doctor's request:

"Now, James, don't you think that new radioisotope scanner written up in the latest journal would be nice to have for our gastrointestinal service? . . . Um . . . just a minute, I seem to detect a slight thrill here. Have you had any episodes of breathlessness or unusually rapid heart beats recently? Well. We must keep an eye on it, mustn't we?"

Under pressures of this type, a strong man can be reduced to a jellyfish. And at the next trustee meeting, that scanner gets approved without a murmur, no matter what the hospital administrator may say.

That is only the beginning. With a new device for screening liver, lung, or brain diseases (the radioisotope scanner), up go the requests for its use. This is encouraged now by the administrator because he can at least begin to amortize its cost and the medical staff can justify the installation.

With more patients screened by the new gadget, more abnormalities will be suspected. This in turn will justify more hospitalization, further laboratory testing, more drugs, and possible surgery—which could have been avoided. Need is expanding with the availability of manpower and machines to satisfy it, just as it did at Duke University Medical Center.

This may not be all bad. Where there are real needs, there is little question that they should be met, depending on other priorities. The trouble is that the decision to expand the service or to buy the equipment is made on the basis of prestige or because of the unquestioned wishes of the medical staff. Rarely, if ever, is it made on the basis of a demonstrable need in the community.

Dr. John Knowles—who as a former hospital administrator has had to work with a board of trustees at the Massachusetts General Hospital—has said that the hospital trustee system is anachronistic and needs reviewing.

There are signs that hospitals are beginning to be less autocratic in their attitude towards their customers—the patients. At the University of Michigan Hospital in Ann Arbor, for example, a service called "Healthy Line" was installed in June of 1972. It enables patients to get information and assistance on any problems they have encountered during the course of their care at the hospital.

They simply dial a phone number, any time of the day or night, relate their problem and where they can be reached and the hospital staff say they will get to work on it right away. "I am convinced that more has to be done in hospitals to help the patient who gets caught in the system," says Louis Graff, director of health science relations at the University Medical Center who thought up the idea.

This is only one hospital and part of a modern, forward-looking medical center at that—a far cry from Blackstone Hospital. But it is a sign of the times and is reflected at the national level by a position taken by the Joint Commission on Accreditation of Hospitals—the body that sets standards for hospital and surgical practice. The organization recently brought out a "Bill of Rights" for patients in accredited hospitals:

"Equitable and humane treatment at all times and under all circumstances is a right," the Commission declared. "It is the duty of everyone involved in taking care of a patient to recognize and respect his individuality and his dignity. . . . In addition, the patient has the right to be informed as to the nature and purpose of any technical procedures which are to be performed upon him, as well as to know by whom such procedures are to be carried out. . . . The patient has the right to communicate with those responsible for his care, and to receive from them adequate information concerning the nature and extent of his medical problem, the planned course of treatment, and the prognosis."

XI

What Health Services Don't Do —Keep You Healthy

The ambulance's siren screams; its red lights flash; by the operating-room table the surgeon stands, masked and gowned:

"Quick, nurse, the DeBakey clamp and a number four Fogarty."

This is the popular picture of American medicine at work. Crisis met with cool competence. It sounds great. But it's no way to provide health care.

Indeed, it's the basic problem with our health services, and, probably, those of any western country. As a prominent British doctor once told us, "The difficulty with our National Health Service is that it isn't a health service at all, it's a National Sick Service."

Modern medicine is geared to dealing with disease, not to preventing it. This is not only poor medicine, which is bad enough, it's also poor economics. It is one reason why we are in today's spiral of rising costs for health services.

The hospital, more than any other medical institution, epitomizes this situation. It stands aloof, like a maitre d' with menus in hand, at the velvet rope of a luxury restaurant. Indeed, the hospital bears about the same relationship to the problem of disease as such restaurants do to the problem of malnutrition. The restaurant is glad to provide you with a gourmet meal, particularly if you have a reservation and a credit card. But with the coffee comes the check and once *that* matter is settled, departure is imminent. "But do dine with us again some other time!"

Health care experts have noted repeatedly that none of the really useful improvements in national health have occurred inside the hospital. What is broadly known as public health has done far more to eradicate the impact of disease than have miracle drugs or surgical procedures.

It goes back to John Snow, who in 1849, successfully prevented cholera from spreading in London by removing the handle of the Broad Street pump. It goes further back, to Edward Jenner who, in 1796, found the value of immunization against smallpox. And you can think back to the days of polio, which are within the living memory of anyone over twenty-five. If it had not been for the development of a vaccine against polio (a research achievement) and its widespread use (a public health achievement), hospitals would still be treating polio, although maybe with more efficient respirators. As far as influencing the spread of the virus in the community, the effect of the hospital would be nil.

There are signs that the modern hospital realizes this. Some few of them are beginning to branch out and put down roots in the communities they serve, in an attempt to really tackle the causes of the problems brought to them and to treat these problems instead of being satisfied with managing the patient's symptoms.

Neighborhood community health centers, for example,

have been established in many cities. Tufts University School of Medicine in Boston has opened encouragingly useful medical, health, and nutritional services both in an urban setting, in Boston, and in a rural setting, in Mississippi.

Other major medical centers are taking similar if less dramatic steps, such as opening satellite clinics, in effect extramural outpatient departments, which should in time combat the actual causes of disease in the community.

But in the smaller community hospitals, this process has, to all practical purposes, hardly started.

Perhaps it is not fair to blame the hospital for this attitude. It really starts with the physician, or, to come right down to it, with the patient.

Traditionally, you see a doctor when you are sick. You then expect him to cure you. What he actually does is to tide you over with painkillers, tranquilizers, or with symptom-relieving drugs until you feel better. Your recuperative process is one that he has little real control over—although it is what pulls you through over 50 percent of the time.

Admittedly, this is something of an exaggeration. Doctors and hospitals are not complete nihilists, nor are they quite as powerless, especially today. In 1970, for example, a little boy in Ohio who was bitten by a rabid bat was successfully treated in a hospital and ultimately made a complete recovery—the first known recovery from rabies ever reported. If he had not been put into hospital and given heroic supportive measures to keep his heart and respiration going as well as drugs and other procedures, he would certainly have died. In less dramatic circumstances, involving many well-established conditions (sometimes even when the cause of the illness remains elusive), this same situation happens in every large hospital.

But, by and large, doctors and hospitals treat people who are sick and return them to the same world where they contracted the sickness and where, all too often, they get sick again. Our point is that by far the largest costs in medical care are based on treating the sick, not in preventing disease. While western doctors are investigating acupuncture in Chinese medicine, they might do well to look into that ancient Oriental practice of paying a physician to keep you well, and not paying him if you became sick, because this represented a failure of care on his part.

Certain health insurance plans—such as the Kaiser Plan in California and Group Health in Washington, D.C.—call for a set pre-payment from the patient and, in return, supply whatever services he or she needs. This is the start of true insurance against illness—although, unfortunately, the physicians working for these groups still tend to think along the more traditional lines of simply treating sickness.

Medical checkups, increasingly popular today, are a step in the right direction. Unfortunately, these measures are all too often discouraged by health insurance providers. Many plans do not underwrite office visits or diagnostic tests if these are made on an outpatient basis. So these insurers encourage excess expenditure by forcing the physician to send the patient to hospital for these tests, which are then reimbursed. This attitude is changing, but it has taken a long time.

Perhaps the best example of where this emphasis has led us are the unoccupied hospital beds. The American Hospital Association estimates that one-fifth of the nation's hospital beds are unused. This amounts annually to 186,560 idle beds at a cost to the health consumer of $3.6 billion. Elliot Richardson, Secretary of the Department of Health, Education, and Welfare, told the Hospital Association at their annual meeting in 1971 that Americans could save $10 billion in hospital construction costs alone if hospital admissions were reduced by 10 percent, length of stay cut by one day, and occupancy rates raised to 90 percent—a logically attainable goal.

In Massachusetts, to cite one well-populated state, unneeded hospital beds hang like a millstone around the public's neck. One-quarter of the hospital beds in the Boston area are unused. It costs taxpayers $65,000 a day, or $455,000 a week, or $24 million a year to maintain these unfilled beds. This sum is twice the amount needed to finance all of Boston's twenty-seven neighborhood health clinics for a year. It could set up eight Community Health Plans serving the total health needs, on an outpatient basis, for 150,000 people. Indeed, it would finance a year of bi-monthly visits to a doctor by every man, woman, and child in Roxbury, a Boston inner city district. Viewed another way, this sum would pay 20 percent of the $124 million that hospitals have received from Medicaid during the fiscal year 1971.

There are signs that some semblance of sanity is beginning to make an impact on this situation. New York, California, and Rhode Island have all passed legislation to regulate the funding of expanded health facilities. Two similar bills are pending in the Massachusetts legislature, requiring a certificate of need by any hospital before it is permitted to expand the number of beds it provides.

In New York, legislation has prevented the setting up of several unnecessary health projects, and better control and management of health facilities has effectively reduced the number of cases sent to hospital. Results are promising. Blue Cross subscribers in New York City are now hospitalized at the rate of 701 hospital days per thousand subscribers, while in Massachusetts, with as yet no control over the provision of health facilities, the rate is 968 hospital days per thousand.

In short, legislation of this type is forcing health providers to think in terms of regional health resources instead of parochial institutional interests.

The hospitals, having enlarged their bed capacity and outfitted themselves with modern medical gadgetry, have had to figure out ways to keep all this capital occupied—or amortized, as accountants say. Nowhere is this more apparent than in the pressure a hospital may exert to ensure maximum utilization of beds, laboratory facilities, X-rays, and operating room equipment—even when they may not really be needed. Enoch Powell, Britain's former Minister of Health, has said that "there is virtually no limit to the amount of medical care an individual is capable of absorbing." The American health economics writer, Jay Nelson Tuck, adds that "there is no way of measuring how many medically unnecessary tests are given or how much unnecessary care is rendered . . . but it is generally agreed that the amount is not trivial."

The extent of this type of overuse has been put at between 5 and 10 percent in New York City—an extremely conservative estimate. If so, it is certainly much higher in less well-controlled communities. There are committees that are supposed to control over-utilization of hospital days, but they do not function effectively since there is no control over the over-utilization of laboratory tests, X-rays, and medical and surgical treatments.

Under the guise of better medical care, hospitals have instituted rules which tend to keep the hospital services and

equipment fully employed rather than the patient healthy—
as we saw in the case of Mrs. Nancy G., who, like every
other patient at Blackstone Hospital, was required to have a
chest X-ray, an electrocardiogram, and blood and urine
tests, although she was only going in to have two wisdom
teeth removed.

XII

How the Medical Care Merchants Cheat the Patient

In trying to protect yourself against unscrupulous medical practitioners, it may be helpful to have some knowledge of the sorts of abuses to which you may be exposed. So we have taken some examples, broken down by specialties, of the way we found medicine and surgery practised at the Blackstone Community Hospital. It is possible that not every suburb is as badly served as is Blackstone's but in many respects it is typical, and our review is intended as a guide to help you, the patient, distinguish good medical care from bad.

In many actual instances, it might be impossible for you, as an individual purchaser of health care, to do anything about the problems of local health care delivery, and you may not even be aware that problems exist, so carefully do some medical practitioners cover their tracks. But, once alerted to the types of abuses, even if individual action to protect yourself is impossible, you can consider supporting state or even federal regulations aimed at reducing them. This could ultimately mean better health services for everyone.

GENERAL PRACTITIONERS

The good general practitioner is the patient's first line of defence in ensuring proper medical care. But there are some GP's who serve as mere traffic officers, directing patients to different specialists. For this, the doctor is possibly given either a direct kickback, such as a percentage of the specialist's fee, or he may get preferential treatment from the chiefs of the medical and surgical departments at the local hospital. In these circumstances, the decision for specialist care is not made on the basis of the patient's needs, and the choice of specialist is not made on the basis of competence but rather on whether or not the referring GP can expect to receive any personal benefit from referring the patient.

We found a number of instances of such improper practices at Blackstone. Although they would have been virtually impossible to prove, everyone knew they existed.

We also found GP's assisting at complicated surgery. It was not clear what they were doing at these operations because they did not have the required skill to be of any help. They were even in the way, and we found instances where the GP's themselves realized this and merely put in a token appearance in the operating room for a few minutes, during surgery. They still received a fee for this "assistance," however—estimated at 15 to 30 percent of the surgeon's bill.

The same referring doctor also frequently followed up on the patient after the surgery, with the excuse that he was there to deal with possible complications or providing medical support—for which of course, he received additional payment. This practice is reimbursed, and therefore condoned, by the health insurance carriers.

Another way that Blackstone has managed to keep its

staff busy is providing "care" for the elderly under Medicare. We found that more than half of the patients with chronic illnesses in Blackstone Hospital were over 65 years of age. They had been admitted by their GP from nursing homes for laboratory and other examinations. It is virtually axiomatic that in patients of advanced age there are bound to be several medical problems. This permits the GP to play favorites with the various specialists in the hospital by requesting multiple consultations on every patient.

For example, perhaps the patient has an acute condition, pneumonia, for which he is admitted to the hospital. But he may also have diabetes, high blood pressure, and underlying coronary artery disease. Once the pneumonia is dealt with and the patient's condition stabilized, it is not difficult for the referring physician to request consultation from any of the specialists on the staff on one or other of the chronic ailments that his elderly patient suffers from.

The benefits of this practice to the GP are two-fold. He receives payment for looking after the patient, and he is able to dispense patronage to the specialists in the hospital in the form of a consultation. The patient's interests are forgotten. He has become an innocent chattel to be shunted from physician to specialist and back again, in the name of good medical care.

This does not mean that every patient at Blackstone was treated in this manner, but we do emphasize that a large number were plainly not in need of the multiple consultations that they received while in the hospital. Their chronic problems were not improved as a result.

This corrupting effect of economic incentive makes itself felt in small aspects of medical practice as well as the large ones. For example, Blue Shield, Medicare, and other insurance carriers have agreed to pay $5 per suture in the repair of any minor cuts that require stitching. Thus a one-inch long laceration which could be satisfactorily closed by inserting two or three stitches in fact receives perhaps as many as six—thus doubling the cost of the procedure.

INTERNISTS

The internist has been called the modern GP. He has usually had some specialized medical training for a period of two or three years as a resident after his internship. However, not more than half the internists who describe themselves as such are in fact certified by the American Board of Internal Medicine.

At Blackstone Hospital, we found only one-third of the internists were board certified. The rest had only short periods of training in this specialty and had not passed their board examinations. Nevertheless, these unqualified men were taking on complicated medical problems, attending heart patients in the intensive care unit, and supervising the treatment of patients with serious neurological and pulmonary diseases. Fees for these services were charged as if they had been performed by fully qualified internists. We also found instances where costs to the patient were inflated by the ordering of unnecessary laboratory tests and undue prolongation of hospitalization or treatment. Perhaps this reflected the physicians' own uncertainty due to their lack of experience or qualifications. The end result was to give the patient poorer service at a higher cost.

GENERAL SURGEONS

At Blackstone Hospital, we found non-surgically-qualified

physicians doing major surgery and highly specialized procedures such as chest, heart and blood vessel surgery.

There was also a great deal of unnecessary surgery, including hernia repairs, varicose vein stripping, appendectomies, and gall bladder removal. (Five million gall bladders
are removed every year in the United States and how many
of these could have been left in the patients has not been estimated.) Up to 30 percent of the organs removed at the
Blackstone Hospital were reported as normal by the pathologist. Although there are times when removal of normal tissue is justified, this percentage is on the high side.

One surgeon performed appendectomies under the diagnosis of "traction appendicitis." We could find no satisfactory explanation of this alleged pathological condition and
could only conclude that he had created it himself. There
was no satisfactory inquiry into these operations or any
record of action taken against this surgeon by the hospital's
tissue committee.

Among the many instances of inadequate procedures attempted by improperly qualified or inexperienced men, one
case stood out because of the peculiarly wanton attitude of
the surgeon. It concerned an automobile accident victim
with a serious head injury. The patient had evidence of brain
damage. A tracheotomy was performed to let the patient
have oxygen. At the end of a week, the tracheotomy had
started to bleed, and in an effort to control this, the surgeon
opened the patient's chest by a split-sternal incision, and
then proceeded to tie off all the arteries supplying blood to
the brain. This left the patient with absolutely no chance of
survival. What is even more extraordinary is that this "surgery" was performed at the bedside without, it seems, any
anesthesia, proper lighting, or other ancillary facilities. As-

sisting at the procedure was an obstetrician! To cap it all, the surgeon himself became the chief of surgery at the hospital—surely the one man who should have been setting an example on the proper way to manage patients. Apparently, he failed to appreciate the nature of the problems he faced and made no effort to find proper help.

ORTHOPEDIC SURGEONS

There was a great deal of unnecessary spinal disc surgery. In at least half the cases at Blackstone Hospital, it was not clearly indicated. A number of orthopedic surgeons in the area also provided physiotherapy and employed full-time physiotherapists in their own offices. This surely is a conflict of interest, like physicians owning pharmacies and dispensing drugs—practices not permitted in many states.

EAR, NOSE, AND THROAT SPECIALISTS

In some 70 percent of that commonest ENT procedure, the tonsillectomy and adenoidectomy, there seemed no adequate indication for the operation. This bears out findings made in other parts of the country and written up in the medical literature. In about half the specimens removed at the Blackstone Hospital, the tonsils were enlarged rather than diseased. There also appeared to be an excessive number of operations for deviated septum of the nose.

UROLOGISTS

Although urinary tract problems tend to occur with greater frequency in the elderly, at Blackstone Hospital, they seemed to be treated radically rather than conservatively. For example, there were a large number of operations for removal of the prostate gland in patients who did not have any urinary tract obstruction. It is normal for the prostrate to be enlarged in the elderly, and although this must be watched for signs of malignancy, there is little need for the gland's removal merely because it is enlarged.

Then there were an inordinate number of cystoscopies (bladder examinations) and meatotomies (surgical widening of the external urinary tract). Cystoscopy carries the risk of urinary tract infection and potential damage to the kidney. Meatotomy is widely regarded these days as unnecessary. In any event, neither procedure should be routine, as seemed to be the case at Blackstone.

We concluded that approximately two-thirds of the urological procedures at this hospital were unnecessary.

ANESTHESIOLOGISTS

In 80 percent of the surgical operations at Blackstone Hospital, we found the anesthetic was given by a nurse anesthetist, not by the staff anesthesiologist. In a disproportionate number of the more serious operations, the nurse anesthetist was on duty and not the anesthesiologist—who was an MD. However, this reduced attention was not reflected in the fee for these services. The patient was billed for the full amount regardless of whether the professionally qualified anesthesiologist was on the job or not.

There were also frequent occasions—when called upon for help with emergency surgery—the staff anesthesiologist refused flatly to be present.

OBSTETRICIANS AND GYNECOLOGISTS

Up to 40 percent of the hysterectomies performed at Blackstone Hospital were performed without apparent reason, and there was no abnormality at all in 25 percent of the cases. This is slightly higher than the national U.S. average for unnecessary hysterectomy. Most authorities put the figure at 33 percent—that is, one out of three hysterectomies did not need to be done.

There were two particularly glaring examples at Blackstone. One surgeon reported that in eight consecutive hysterectomies the uterus was enlarged, yet at operation and in later examination of the tissue by the pathologist, the organ was found to be of normal size. In the second instance, a gynecologist performed five hysterectomies and all the tissues proved to be normal. It was possibly no accident that, at the time, his close friend the chief of surgery was chairman of the hospital's tissue committee which supposedly prevents this kind of unnecessary surgery.

LABORATORY SERVICES

As much as 90 percent of the laboratory work reported negative findings or simply confirmed or duplicated other tests. Many laboratory tests are useful in selected cases but their wholesale application to every patient who comes into the hospital just increases the cost to that patient.

PATHOLOGY SERVICES

The chief of pathology at Blackstone Hospital was six months behind in reporting his autopsy specimens. One reason was that he engaged in other work outside the hospital and also ran a private pathology laboratory. Frozen tissue sections were poorly prepared, with the result that diagnoses were frequently inaccurate. For example, in one series of specimens taken from a mass in the chest of a patient, the pathologist reported that they were malignant. Yet when studied later, they turned out to be benign. Other examples of reverse misleading diagnoses based on frozen sections were found. These are particularly important because a decision concerning the treatment of the patient is often made on the basis of a report on the frozen section, done while the patient is on the operating table.

RADIOLOGISTS

As in the laboratory services, we found many unnecessary and repetitive X-rays and radiological tests performed at Blackstone Hospital. There were numerous instances of arteriograms done on the blood vessels of both legs when only the vessels on one leg had been requested. Since this procedure is not without hazard, this seemed unwise, quite apart from the expense, to subject the patient to it, particularly when it was not indicated.

There was also enthusiasm for far-fetched tests in otherwise clear-cut cases. We found one patient with ovarian cancer where the disease had, by the time of the test we are discussing, spread to the liver with abdominal distension from ascitic fluid. Nevertheless, the patient was subjected to an ovarian arteriography—a process used to delineate the presence of the blood vessels, if any, leading to the tumorous area—and diagnostic of ovarian cancer. Here it seemed redundant. Furthermore, the test led to complications for this patient. As a result of injury to the blood vessel used for the injection of radio-opaque dye, her femoral artery became blocked and three more operations were required to reestablish a satisfactory blood flow to the leg. The patient died two months later, her life probably shortened by this over-enthusiastic use of a modern diagnostic tool. Certainly it added to the misery of her last remaining months.

If you, or a member of your family such as an elderly

parent, has to be hospitalized in an institution such as Blackstone, how can you be sure that the specialist you employ really is a specialist?

You look him up in the *Directory of Medical Specialists,* which you'll find in the public library. This book makes interesting reading in the light of what we have seen at the Blackstone Hospital. For example, the 1970 edition lists some 108,000 board certified specialists in active practice. This is only about one-third of the total number of practicing physicians in the U.S.A. However, as we noted earlier, 80 percent of the physicians in this country describe themselves as practicing some sort of medical or surgical specialty. This means that some 40 percent of those doctors who claim to be specialists are in fact misrepresenting themselves and hoodwinking the consumer of medical care into paying more for their services than they should. Specialists charge more than general practitioners for their services.

Consider these figures published in the *Journal of the American Medical Association.* The number of board-certified specialists in anesthesia is only half the total number of those physicians who actually practice anesthesiology in the U.S.; among those who call themselves internists only 45 percent are board certified; of psychiatrists only 48 percent are board certified; of the surgical sub-specialty colon and rectal surgery only 55 percent are board certified; finally, only 58 percent of the practicing urologists are board certified.

The true specialist has to undergo a required number of progressively graded years of approved residency training in a major teaching hospital. He has then to take extensive oral and written examinations supervised by these specialty boards. Upon satisfactorily passing these examinations, he receives a certificate that he has been admitted to the specialty in question, and he is then listed in the Directory of Medical Specialists, where you can find his name.

Many non-qualified "specialists" claim varying years of experience or training in their specialty and indeed they may have had some exposure to the field they claim. But the fact remains that they are not board certified and should not be allowed to practice as specialists and charge specialist fees any more than a person who has spent a couple of years at a medical school should be allowed to practice as a doctor. Some physicians who fail to pass their specialty examinations nevertheless go on to describe themselves as specialists, and this should not be permitted.

Third party insurers, both public and private, unfortunately compound the issue by paying specialist fees for services rended by improperly qualified practitioners. If they adopted the principle of paying only for board-certified physicians when such a fee is charged, there would be a considerable saving in medical costs, and less surgery and complicated procedures undertaken by these non-specialists.

This in turn might have a salutary effect on the number of malpractice suits that so frequently plague physicians and surgeons today. Surgical and medical procedures performed by insufficiently qualified men tend to be accompanied by more complications and poor results. If these men were not permitted to undertake such procedures in the first place, it might reduce the cost of malpractice insurance—a heavy burden on doctors and one that is in turn passed on to the patient in the form of higher fees.

Don't assume that because a doctor is in partnership with a properly certified board specialist that he is necessarily qualified in that particular specialty. Recently various groups of medical and surgical specialists have formed themselves into corporations or associations, such as obstetric and gynecological associates, surgical associates, and so forth. Sometimes three or four doctors will set up specialist practice together under a corporate name even though only one or perhaps two of them is board certified. All the members of the corporation receive the full specialists' fee for their services from the health insurance carriers just as if they were in fact board-certified specialists.

Frequently, three or four of these associates may see the same patient on different occasions. And each submits his own separate consultation fee. It has become almost routine for some associations deliberately to arrange such double payments under the guise of providing coverage when the specialist who first saw the patient happens to have the day off.

Do not assume either that because you may be seeing several specialists in such an association that you are therefore receiving an independent consultation. Such physicians, working together as they do, are likely to confirm each other's findings and mutually agree on the recommendations to be followed.

Not all group practices are conducive to good medicine. One physician we know joined a group expecting that he would be able to practice better medicine than he could have done in solo practice. But at the end of his first year, he was called in by the group's accountant and informed that he was not pulling his financial weight. He would just have to see more patients in the future.

The man resigned and joined the Veterans Administration as a medical officer. There he is a government servant and is paid a salary. He doesn't make as much money as his former partners but he practices what he considers good medicine. And, as he says, "That's what I went to medical school for."

There seems no good reason why government insurance plans like Medicare or private health insurance companies should make payments for specialist services to non-board-certified specialists. Indeed, the medical services of the armed forces do not grant a full specialist grading to a non-specialist.

If government insurers and other health carriers would adopt this attitude of only recognizing the board-certified man as a specialist, the result would be an enormous saving to the public in medical costs and the elimination of many unnecessary services performed by inadequately qualified individuals. And it would make medical care much safer for the patient.

XIII

Health Insurance: The Way it Affects the Care You Get

SCENE I: Corridor in a hospital. Two physicians are talking.

First Physician

(a young man): Do you think all these additional tests are really necessary? The indications are pretty clear, the SGOT level is up and . . . well, just take a look at him.

Second Physician

(a consultant): Maybe so, but let's do them all anyway. I'd particularly like to see if the lab can spot Australia antigen in the serum. Besides it looks good on the chart for the utilization committee. And, remember, his insurance will cover it.

SCENE II: Doctor's office. Doctor and patient are talking.

Doctor: My examination shows that you have a deviated septum of the nose. I recommend strongly that you have it operated on immediately. I'll make the necessary arrangements with the hospital.

123

Patient

(male, fortyish,

hesitant): Well, I don't know . . . it doesn't seem to be
bothering me much.

Doctor: You don't want the condition to get worse, do
you? Come now, after all your insurance company will pay for it.

Patient

(resignedly): I suppose so, if you say so, doctor. . . .

So the insurance will pay for it all.

Right? Wrong.

No matter how well covered you think you are, it's you,
the consumer, who pays in the end. Indeed, short of some totally comprehensive coverage, your health insurance plan
probably will not meet all your medical cost.

These two scenes illustrate some of the things that are
wrong with health insurance plans today. Health insurance
has stimulated needless demands and unnecessary services,
both on the part of the doctor and of the patient. So now insurance coverage for essential medical services is inadequate
for those who really need it.

Comprehensive insurance policies, from the private company's point of view, are very difficult to write, and the
reason is not far to seek.

Private insurance works well against single risks, such as
the chance that you may be involved in an automobile accident, or that your house may burn down. But it is quite unable to provide adequate coverage for life against sickness,
because of the wide variety of diseases and treatments.

So, in order to keep costs down, the private insurance
company restricts the individuals it will insure. It takes only

the "good risks"—and falls back on restrictions, limitations and exclusions as well as other "fine print," which all too often makes its coverage useless to the individual it is supposed to cover.

A reason for this lies in the way health insurance has developed in the United States. Today's consumer would do well to remember that health insurance in this country was first devised to serve the interests of the health providers rather than that of the patients. In the 1930s, at the height of the depression, hospitals had empty beds and unpaid bills. Fortunately, these problems were solved after a group of Dallas public school teachers developed a prepaid program whereby Baylor University Hospital agreed to provide certain health services in exchange for a relatively small periodic payment. With this experience as a guide to premiums and benefits, hospitals began to enroll other groups on the same basis to answer their need for a dependable, regular source of income. Thus the first Blue Cross Association was formed. Similar programs grew rapidly, and by 1971 Blue Cross had 75 million members—38 percent of the population —and was paying out $6.05 billion annually on their behalf.

But basically Blue Cross was set up to serve hospitals, not patients. In the beginning, the hospitals' interest in keeping a stable financial base did not conflict with the consumers' interests, and the Blue Cross service contracts provided quite comprehensive coverage at reasonably low rates. (A service contract entitles the beneficiary to certain specified services as opposed to an insurance plan that provides cash to the individual for part of his expenses.)

As the years passed, the service contract has become the equivalent of a cost-plus contract. The hospitals started telling the Blue Cross what they wanted to charge for services, and the Association paid, without regard to whether these costs represented a fair price for the service rendered or whether the hospital was padding the bill. After all, reasoned the Association, they represented the hospital, not the patient. When costs rose, as they inevitably did, either Blue Cross raised its rates for membership or it reduced the services that it covered. In recent years, it has done both.

The result is that health insurance has become not only more expensive, but less comprehensive. The Blue Cross member is paying more for less.

While Blue Cross was growing during the 1930s, physicians in general took a poor view of prepaid health insurance of any kind. Their words then have a familiar ring to those who have lived through the long fight for Medicare and currently for National Health Insurance.

But by 1938, physicians had begun to realize that third party coverage of medical services was here to stay, and if they wanted it to serve their interest they had better devise a plan of their own. They were assisted to this conclusion by the courts. Organized medicine's resistance to prepaid group practice had resulted in an indictment being brought against the physicians under the Sherman Anti-Trust Act. The physicians lost their case. They were held to be in contravention of the Act by restraining the practice of medicine.

The physicians' response to this was the beginning of Blue Shield—the "doctors' plan"—which in 1971 had 66.6 million subscribers, who gave $2.5 billion in benefits to be paid to physicians for medical and surgical services.

Note that just as Blue Cross was developed to serve the hospital and guarantee that the hospital would be paid for the service it provided, so Blue Shield came into existence for the benefit of the physicians, not the patients. Under

Blue Shield, what the physician is doing is guaranteeing that he will be paid for the service he provides. Whether that service is in fact necessary is not the issue with Blue Shield. Yet if costs of medical care are to be held down, then whether the service is really necessary or not is in fact the central issue. It brings us right back to what we said at the very beginning of this book. Without control of the *quality* of care, we can never control its *cost*.

Incidentally, this long fight that the public has had—and continues to have—with the medical profession over third party health insurance is not without its ironies. While official medicine fought tooth and nail against such plans, once they were in effect the real beneficiary turned out to be the physician, not his patient. Third party insurance has freed the physician to perform what treatment he thinks necessary for his patient with assurance that he will be paid.

Quite apart from the fact that this has had the effect of forcing up the nation's total medical bill, it has also guaranteed the doctor's income in an open-ended manner. Had there been no third party health insurance, such guarantees would have been impossible. Although officially the medical profession was against third party intrusion into health care, nevertheless when it eventually did come about it did so in a manner that virtually assured doctors that if they wished they could become rich men. This is exactly what has happened, as we saw in Chapter VII. Never has so much been reaped by so few for so much obstruction.

With non-profit third party health insurance now established and filling a demand for prepaid health insurance, the private insurance companies, spotting an opportunity to make money, began to move in. They saw the possibilities of being able to sell complete packages of insurance, including life, accident, property, pensions, and so forth, together with health.

However, an insurance company providing protection for its own profit must insure against known risks. When a company insures your automobile or your life, it does so knowing what the chances are that your car will be involved in an accident or what the risk is that you yourself will die next year instead of thirty years from now. This risk is determined by standard actuarial principles.

But the likelihood of expenses arising from sickness is not so precisely determinable by statistical means, because whether the insured person seeks medical attention is not always within his own control or that of his insurance company. Hence, insurance vendors have sought to blunt the possibility that the insured person might use his health insurance unnecessarily by inserting limitations and definitions of what kind of expenses they will pay. They also eliminate coverage for individuals who are known to be high risk cases, such as the elderly and those with a history of chronic illness.

Take the case of Mary Lynn Fletcher, crippled by polio in 1951 when she was five. She told a Senate subcommittee hearing that because she is partially paralyzed below the waist, she could get only restricted health insurance. Health insurance insures only the healthy, she observed and quoted to Senators Philip D. Hart (D. Mich.) and Edward M. Kennedy (D. Mass.) that one insurance company agent told her: "We can't possibly insure you because we would lose money."

Miss Fletcher does have a limited health insurance policy, but it has a restriction which excludes coverage for any disease or injury to the lower extremities.

Insurance companies also exclude entirely such preventive services as out-of-hospital checkups and so forth. Thus private companies cannot provide truly comprehensive health insurance for anyone.

An illustration of how health insurance companies have warped the way the patient receives health care is the well-known fact that treatment and tests given in a hospital get favored coverage over the same therapy given in a doctor's office or a clinic.

As Dr. William MacColl puts it in his book *Group Practice and Prepayment of Medical Care:* "The insurance companies find themselves applying the traditional mechanisms of insurance against specific catastrophes to a completely different problem—that of day-to-day health care, including health maintenance as well as services for disabling illness." They have developed "a veritable avalanche" of policies which have been more often designed with the company than the consumer in mind and, as Dr. MacColl adds, "without a basic understanding of the systems through which health services are delivered to patients."

The health insurers are digging their own grave by not realizing the true nature of what they are insuring against. They discourage people from seeking prepaid medical care in the doctor's office or clinic when disease is in the early stages and when it can be most cheaply and effectively treated, and encourage overuse of hospitalization for procedures that can be handled just as effectively in a doctor's office.

So, in order to stay in business, the health insurance industry has had to either restrict the services it covers or make them extremely expensive to purchase. This situation has now gone so far, that, ironically, it threatens to put the private health insurance companies out of business entirely.

The development of private health insurance has also had its effect on Blue Cross. The private company can provide coverage to a group or an individual on an experience-rated basis—that is, the rates are lower for those who are known to be healthier or less likely to need medical aid than for those likely to become ill. Traditionally, Blue Cross offered its coverage on a community basis. Rates and costs were based on the average experience of the entire community, not just segments of it. In this way high- and low-risk groups received coverage at the same rates.

But when the private companies began offering coverage at much lower rates to more favored groups, Blue Cross was left holding the high-risk groups and soon found itself under heavy economic pressure. This in turn meant the Association either had to resort to deductibles and co-insurance clauses to control costs or they had to follow the line of the commercial companies and discard community rating. Either way, the Blue Cross subscriber lost out.

With insurance coverage sold to different groups at different rates, those who most needed health insurance—the elderly, the sick and unemployed—had to pay the highest premiums. This is simply good insurance business, but it is also another example of how health insurance distorts our real priorities. Dr. MacColl describes it as "socially obnoxious."

In short, competition in the health insurance business has served to benefit primarily those who need such insurance least.

Health insurance by itself has increased the use of physicians' services, hospital, and health facilities in general, as was pointed out many years ago by Odin Anderson of the University of Chicago. Dr. Anderson found that rates for surgery among insured persons were twice that for those who were not insured. This in turn has stimulated an inflation of medical care costs.

Insurance companies are aware of the abuses uncovered by investigations such as Dr. Anderson's, and they have their own figures. They know that when they insure a person he is more likely to seek medical aid under his insurance coverage —or have it thrust upon him by his doctor. So the companies allow for this possibility or "abuse" by increasing their premiums. Higher charges are the result. So the consumer loses again, not only through increased costs for services but through paying higher premiums for those services he does get.

In case the reader assumes that it is only the private insurance companies that fail to provide adequate cost control mechanisms, we should emphasize that *all* health insurance, including government plans such as Medicare and Medicaid, are equally responsible.

Experience with Medicare and Medicaid shows plainly that if and when national health insurance becomes a reality in the United States, costs of health care will continue to mount unless an effective system of cost control is built in.

In the years from 1967 to 1971, the cost of Medicaid has more than doubled and the cost of Medicare has nearly tripled. Most of this increase was fueled by these programs themselves. As Irving J. Lewis of Albert Einstein College of Medicine in New York has pointed out, our medical resources are not unlimited. By pumping money into medical-benefit programs without controlling the services provided under them, the government contributed to the inflation of medical costs. The result is that the cost of hospital care today is three times what it was in 1957 and physicians' fees have risen twice as fast as the consumer price index. In a very real sense the health professional has become wealthy at public expense.

This, however, does not help you with your current problems about health insurance today, although such lessons may be of help in future planning. As a partial answer to your difficulty, we have prepared in the next chapter what we hope will be some helpful hints on health insurance and how to manage the almost inevitable problems that will be involved in settling your medical bills.

XIV

Health Insurance: Trying to Beat the System

As we have just seen, the health insurance companies take your money in the form of premiums, but they cannot exercise much control over the providers of the services you are insured for, so in a desperate attempt to keep down costs, they try to limit your health insurance coverage by writing various kinds of restrictions into their policies. They tackle the problem of costs from the wrong end. They try to restrict you, the consumer, from using your policy at earlier stages in illness when it would be much cheaper to have it treated; and they encourage a health policy's use only when you are sick enough to seek medical attention, when the illness has advanced to the point where it will be much more expensive to treat.

How do you beat this situation? The answer, quite bluntly, is that you can't. You're bound to lose on health insurance.

But that's no reason to despair. Everyone, at some point in life, has to do business under less than ideal conditions. What you can do here is keep your inevitable losses to a minimum while getting your maximum benefits from your

133

health insurance.

You could, for instance, avoid taking out any health insurance at all. But this would be foolhardy. The risks are too great. Even a rich man could end up in debt after a brush with the health profession, as it is run today. Besides, it *is* possible to use existing health plans, even when less than ideal, to pay *some* of your medical bills. And every little bit helps.

Most likely, you have some health insurance coverage through your job or professional association. This is probably the best protection for the price. But unless it is fully comprehensive, providing a broad range of benefits, covering you and your family both at work and during off hours, you may not be completely protected. In this case, you should fill in the gaps with an additional policy. Look for areas where your coverage seems inadequate—or even non-existent. If you can't understand all the fine print, show the policy to some independent authority, such as your accountant or lawyer, to spot restrictions, such as deductibles or co-insurance, and exclusions such as those for pre-existing conditions, or limitations such as those for coverage of mental illness.

Deductibles are amounts which you agree to pay yourself before a claim will be considered. They are similar to clauses in automobile insurance where you agree to pay for damages up to $100 before making any claim. Policies with high deductible clauses are cheaper than those that cover you completely or in which the deductible is only a small, token sum.

Co-insurance is when you agree to pay a percentage of the payable amount under the policy. Thus if the bill comes to $1000 and the deductible is $100 and the co-insurance 25 percent, then the insurance company will only pay $675 of your claim. You pay $325—the $100 deductible and the 25 percent co-insurance.

It is important to make certain whether such limits apply to each claim individually or only within a specific time, such as within a calendar year or other time limit. Generally a time factor is better than a claim factor because insurance companies have been known to break up a single claim into several factors and then apply the deductible and co-insurance clauses to each. This reduces the company's liability but leaves you with a much higher bill to pay yourself.

It is up to you to take stock of your personal situation, for only you can decide what you need and what you can afford. For example, if you have had all the children you want and your family is complete, you should not have to pay for maternity care coverage. Again, don't wait too long before covering yourself. Health insurance is harder to get as you grow older, and the chances of developing diseases are greater. There comes a point in life when you can't get insurance at favorable rates, sometimes not at all.

Seek independent advice from your lawyer or banker before you purchase health insurance. Also, do some comparison shopping with other insurance brokers. There may be lots of holes, from your particular point of view, in the policy you are considering. Only an independent authority, who knows you and your way of life, can help you decide. Whatever you do, don't buy insurance solicited through direct mail or from those heavily advertised plans that promise you large sums in cash should you be hospitalized.

The chances of you ever being able to collect such sums are remote. The companies concerned have admitted this in public hearings held by the New Jersey State Insurance Commission. "If people have other coverage, they don't need these policies. And people who buy such policies as their only health insurance are not being adequately protected," says Pennsylvania's Insurance Commissioner, Herbert S. Denenberg.

The best type of health insurance policies are those that provide clinical services such as prepaid group practice does, or service benefits as Blue Cross and Blue Shield do. The least desirable policies are those that pay cash. In the insanely complex world of health insurance, if you stick to these principles you'll be making the best of a very difficult situation.

In recent months there have been developments in two states that promise to make purchasing health insurance much easier. California and New York have both developed preliminary plans for grading the various elements of health insurance plans in terms of the benefits they offer and the outlays they incur in the form of premiums. The health department in New York State has developed one model and the School of Public Health at the University of California has proposed another.

The California system has been tested against several health insurance plans and has, so its authors say, proved practical. For example, the system showed, as might be expected, that plans with higher premiums scored better than those with lower. But there were some substantial discrepancies between the cost of the plans tested in terms of the premiums they charged and their ultimate rating in terms of benefit to the consumer. One plan with a premium cost of over $40 scored 470 points; whereas two other plans whose premiums cost only $30 to $35 scored 675 and 586 points respectively.

Underlying these systems is the premise that health insurance is purchased by consumers to protect themselves against economic loss caused by illness. Only by establishing a measure of the economic protection that the policy provides can a policy or insurance plan be evaluated on its merits, the proponents of these plans believe.

"Marketing gimmicks and high pressure sales techniques should not determine the selection of a policy," warns Mildred B. Shapiro, director of the Bureau of Economic Analysis of New York's Department of Health, and author of the New York plan. In this plan, a health insurance policy would be graded in such a way that it would reflect accurately the economic protection and the return obtained for the cost of the policy. This would give the purchaser some concrete guide that would help him in deciding between one plan and another.

Meanwhile, the fact that the Blue Cross or other insurance companies may not question hospital bills is no reason why you, the consumer, should not do so. Does a businessman pay a hotel bill without looking it over carefully simply because his employer will, eventually, reimburse him? Hospital bills have an even wider margin for error than hotel bills, so be warned.

Be sure to get itemized hospital bills. You are entitled to see every charge that the hospital makes, and you have every right to question items you do not understand or did not know about. Some hospitals have been known to go to quite extraordinary lengths to inflate their bills. One even charged a patient $10 for "$H_2O$"—assuming, no doubt, that he didn't know what it was. Another family was charged $20 for moving a dead patient from her room to the hospital's morgue. One elderly lady was given a daily EKG—for a daily consideration—although her doctor had not ordered this. Hospitals, notoriously, overcharge for drugs. Remember even aspirin can be billed for as much as 50 cents per dose. Also, if you are given prescriptions to take home, have these filled by your regular pharmacist who, if you have found a good one, might not charge you as much as the hospital. All these items contribute to increasing your overall health care costs.

Every charge that your doctor makes, you must, if possible, discuss with him beforehand. If not, discuss it as soon as possible afterwards. If you yourself are too sick to do so, have some member of your family take the matter up on your behalf. A surgeon may charge you $700 for an operation that under the scale of "usual and customary fees" is only worth $250. Don't pay him until you've established that the additional charges are justified and that your insurance company will pay all of the charges that your policy covers you for.

Recently some help for the beleagured patient and excessive medical charges has been forthcoming from the courts. In two cases in Philadelphia Municipal Court, the judge ruled that a patient need not pay a hospital bill when the hospital's charges are unreasonable. In the other decision, even although the charges were reasonable, the services provided were held not to be necessary for the patient's welfare. In these circumstances the court ruled that the patient could collect the amount of the bill from the doctor who ordered the unnecessary services.

The suits arose when Blue Cross had determined that the services were not needed and refused to pay the hospitals for them. The hospitals sued the patients for the bills.

In the first case the judgment went in favor of the patient when the hospital's attorney failed to provide evidence of the reasonableness of the hospital's charges. In the second case, the court ruled that the attending physician had ordered admission to hospital for tests that "could and should have been performed on an outpatient basis." In view of this, while the patient had to pay the hospital, he could nevertheless collect the amount of the hospital's bill from the doctor who had ordered the admission to hospital.

These are hopeful signs that the patient's rights are at last being respected. But apart from such legal moves, there are new trends in health insurance and health services that almost certainly will make for easier and more reliable methods of handling sickness benefits than is the case today. Some form of governmentally supervised national health insurance—beyond Medicare and Medicaid—is inevitable. As a voter, you can voice your opinion that cost control mechanisms of one type or another be instituted in such plans to stabilize the benefits obtainable from health insurance. Write to your congressman or senator and let him know that as a consumer you are watching the various health insurance bills for safeguards against mounting costs.

Today even the private carriers are talking about cost control moves which a few years ago they would hardly have countenanced. In part it is because they are now beginning to lose money on policies that limit the patient to in-hospital care or place other restrictions on what they will cover. It has not gone without notice that many smaller independent health insurance plans that stress out-of-hospital benefits are not losing as much money as the older plans that emphasize in-hospital care.

Also, individual doctors have in many cases forced insurance companies to recognize that admitting patients to hospitals for outpatient procedures inflates costs unnecessarily and this is to no one's benefit. Some doctors tell insurance companies bluntly that if they pay for an office procedure instead of admitting the patient to a hospital for it, charges will be several times less. Under these circumstances, companies have been known to pay for the office procedure. Do not hesitate to ask your doctor to discuss such matters with your insurance agent should the need arise in your case. If the doctor does not wish to do this, then perhaps you should take a second look at him and check out whatever he wants to do for you with another authority.

At present, the most comprehensive health insurance available—and even that is far from perfect—is provided by the prepaid, consumer-controlled plans like the Health Insurance Plan of New York, Group Health Insurance of New York and New Jersey, Group Health Association of Washington, D.C., and the Group Health Cooperative of Puget Sound. There are also provider-controlled prepaid plans such as the Ross-Loos Medical Group of Los Angeles, the San Joaquin County Medical Foundation in California, and the Kaiser Foundation Health plan. This last started during the depression years and burgeoned during World War II. Originally it was an industrial prepaid health program for Kaiser Industry employees, but it has now grown into a vast network of community hospitals, clinics, and medical groups with over two million members. Besides California, where the Kaiser Plan originated, there are now Kaiser groups in Washington, Oregon, and Hawaii, as well as Cleveland and Denver. These health delivery systems have already reduced hospitalization rates and markedly cut the number of unnecessary operations in areas such as tonsillectomies.

Then there are plans controlled by labor or management such as the United Mineworkers Welfare and Retirement Fund and other health and welfare funds in many of our major cities. Usually the labor-controlled plans have the advantage of having a union lawyer available to take legal action if the insured individual fails to receive the services to which he is entitled.

Finally, there are some 1,800 private commercial companies that write health insurance on an individual or group basis. Individual health insurance policies are frequently very inefficient. By their own admission, the companies who write health insurance need forty-six cents out of every dollar to administer an individual health insurance policy—and even then they claim they don't make a profit!

For the sake of completeness we should also mention the two relatively new government health plans, Medicare and Medicaid. Medicare is health insurance for the aged. It provides better benefits than any existing private health insurance plan for this age group. Virtually the entire population in the United States over the age of 65 receiving Social Security benefits—some 20 million people—are protected by the hospital part of Medicare, Part A; some 95 percent—over 19 million people—are voluntarily enrolled in the medical insurance part of Medicare, Part B. Approximately 90 percent of the payments in Part B of Medicare settle doctors' bills.

Medicaid is a totally different bird. It is a public assistance program which took over the former categorical welfare programs involving medical care formerly provided by the states. There is an income eligibility formula or means test applied to those who seek benefits from it. Medicare is government-financed health insurance. Medicaid is welfare. In the difference lies the promise of the one and the problems of the other.

Although federal grants under Medicaid provide more than four dollars in five of its cost, the fiscal impact, according to Irving Lewis of Albert Einstein College of Medicine in New York, has been "close to disastrous." State and local spending for medical assistance rose from $764 million in 1965 to $2.3 billion in 1969.

This has resulted in state legislators and administrators cutting back the benefits and reducing the number of eligible people for Medicaid—mainly by reducing the income level at which benefits can be obtained. The result is, as Dr. Lewis notes, that Medicaid reaches only 15 million of the 30 to 40 million people who could be covered. As the government's Task Force on Medicaid has put it: "The promise of Medicaid, that some care at least would be available to all who need it, has vanished into the obscurity of state determination of eligibility and the limitation of state resources."

As we watch the growth and development of health insurance, not the least fascinating is the application this may have to other aspects of our society besides the providing of better medical care.

In most simple market place exchanges, the interest of the purchaser is also in the interest of the provider, at least for the purposes of immediate business. A grocer will not knowingly sell you bad apples or a supplier give you short measure, because they want your business on a repeat basis. The profit in such transactions, in other words, is not solely obtained on a single transaction.

But in medicine, and in many other transactions of modern life, the interest of those who provide the services are not the same as those of the consumers who purchase them. One good example is public transportation. The value of such service is not measurable simply in terms of financial profit to the provider.

We are, today, feeling our way gingerly toward a new type

of economic measurement in which the immediate cash profit may be less beneficial to the community in general than
the service that is provided, therefore it has to be looked at
in other than traditional ways.

We believe that medicine, with its tradition of service to
the well-being of man, is—as the present debates over medical care show—becoming one of the leaders in this as yet
embryonic realization, the full extent of which we are only
beginning to grasp. How society handles problems of this nature in all walks of life, not just in medical care, will make
for some very exciting developments in the coming years.

XV

The Doctor-Watchers—Peer Review and Quality Control

Up to now, this book has been mainly concerned with what you, the patient, can do directly to assure yourself of better health care. We turn now to the larger picture—the ways that doctors and the health care system could be regulated to provide the best services to your community.

The word "regulation" is as a red flag to a bull to many physicians. They see regulation as the dead hand of bureaucracy interfering with the way they practice medicine and especially the hallowed doctor-patient relationship. Such physicians will try to tell you that the end result would be poor medical care.

Install regulations, such individuals say, and the doctor will be unable to do things the way he, as a professional, thinks they should be done for the patient's benefit. They say he will be controlled by some faceless bureaucrat with a schedule of treatments in one hand and a scale of charges in the other.

Don't be fooled by this ploy. It has not happened in countries where such regulations have been in force for many years.

Moreover, in the United States one of the most carefully regulated practices of medicine and surgery is provided by the military services. Yet these are so good that members of Congress, justices of the Supreme Court, even the president and his family regularly make use of them. As part of the military establishment, doctors are on salary, thus they are relieved of the economic motivation to prescribe expensive treatment. Moreover, their work is carefully supervised by senior, and presumably more experienced, medical officers.

Before going on to discuss specific ways that non-military physicians could be effectively regulated and medical abuses reduced to a minimum, let us look at the medical profession's own method of policing and see how satisfactory it is —or rather, how unsatisfactory.

Attempted regulation of physicians is as old as medicine itself. The Code of Hammurabi describes the punishment inflicted on a bad surgeon—he had his hand cut off. Certainly, the leaders in medicine have long recognized the need to keep the less scrupulous members of their profession under control; even, on occasion, to remove them from active practice. One way of keeping the standards high is to prevent undesirable characters from entering the profession at all. Medical schools do this by developing a very careful system of admission and screening. Once a man or woman starts training in patient care, there is a gradual system of progress towards more responsibility, each step supervised by senior doctors.

Further, when a physician leaves medical school and goes out to practice medicine, the professional specialists' associations to which he belongs exercise some control over his activities. Even the family physician these days has his own association, and he is encouraged and sometimes required to attend educational programs to be sure he keeps abreast of medical developments. However, such organizations are by their nature self-regulatory. It is a case of one fellow professional regulating another, and the tendency, except in the most blatant cases, is to do nothing.

In this country, the recognition of the need to standardize the quality of medical care goes back to just before World War I, when a Massachusetts surgeon, Dr. Ernest A. Codman, of Harvard Medical School, urged the medical profession and hospital administrators to make public all the results of the treatment they gave their patients. In other words, he was suggesting that the profession obtain the information necessary to arrive at some valid conclusions about the *quality* of medical care. Dr. Codman caused such a furor among his fellow surgeons that he was ultimately thrown off the Harvard medical faculty, and he died a bitter man.

Today, almost sixty years later, his objective has still not been achieved. It is extraordinarily difficult and often impossible for a lay person—and sometimes even for a professional medical man—to find out what actually happens to a patient in a hospital.

About twenty years ago, as it became apparent that patients were being increasingly exposed to serious abuses, and along with the development of health insurance plans which required some sort of accountability, the American medical profession came up with a system of reviewing their own work. Committees were set up within the hospitals to review specimens of tissue removed during surgery, to make sure that these did, in fact come from diseased organs. If they did not, and the organ had been removed, the surgeon had to justify his actions. He had to give the committee some good reason for having operated on the patient. Similar committees were formed to review the work of other individual hospital departments in an attempt to keep some sort of check on the standard of medicine practiced there. Where such efforts are vigorously pursued, they do reduce unnecessary surgery markedly and they do improve the quality of care.

The members of these committees are physicians and surgeons with experience similar to that of those whose work they investigate. Thus the system came to be called *peer review*—a second look at the work done by other members of the profession, the man's peers. Peer review serves a useful educational function for doctors. It can act as sort of overseer or pressure on medical practice, keeping procedures and treatments within the bounds of what would be considered right in the circumstances. Such a review is similar to the relationship between a master and an apprentice or between the senior and junior man in any profession.

However, within the last few years, this system of self-regulation has exhibited weaknesses, and new proposals are being put forth to revise and modify the present system. The pressure to improve peer review comes from two sources, and for two reasons. One is the increasing complexity of modern medicine (which the doctors well realize); the other is the rising costs of medical care, which today are borne more and more by health insurance agencies. Over half the health care budget in the U.S. is paid for by insurance plans of one type or another. These insurance carriers, with more than 70 million subscribers, increasingly demand more cost and quality control. Peer review is supposed to provide this.

Peer review aims at several things. First, it attempts, through its review of fees, to keep costs down, or at least to identify them. If a physician charges more than the going rate for a particular treatment, the review committee can politely ask him to explain why. In this way, it is hoped that charges for health care will not soar beyond reason.

Secondly, the peer review system tries to insure that the physician conducts himself according to agreed professional and ethical standards, both medically and fiscally, so that the interests of doctor and patient are both served.

Thirdly, peer review is a useful method for letting the public feel reassured that physicians in general are concerned about their patients and about the quality and cost of health services.

This does not mean that peer review committees will report to the public what they have done and why, as, for example, an appellate court would do when handing down a decision. But the supporters of peer review say they believe the actual existence of these committees is an indication of the concern the profession has for the patient.

A recent attempt to improve the peer review system involves the formation of what are known as health care foundations. Sponsored by state medical societies, these have now been started in several states. These foundations have developed treatment guidelines, or profiles, as they call them, for the managing of various diseases, as well as fee schedules for their application.

An insurance claim is screened against this profile, which has been built up through study of comparable cases, e.g., so many hospital days are considered standard for a particular procedure or so many treatment visits are required after a particular operation. If the claim is for more than the usual amount of therapy, then it is referred for review first by a physician and then by the peer review board.

The system has worked well in many states, saving considerable sums in overcharges and other excessive expenditures,
but it is far from perfect. For one thing, it is not clear how
unnecessary surgery is handled under this system. The patient may not have been hospitalized for any excessive
period, the surgeon's bill may be reasonable—but what if the
surgery was not needed at all?

The other difficulty is that not all cases call for identical
treatment, and procedures are constantly changing. The profile guidelines tend to reflect the prevailing practice of the
majority of the physicians in the state, regardless of whether
this practice is the best or the most up-to-date.

Also, peer review may serve a useful educational function
for the physician who is prepared to learn, but if it is to
work, it must also discipline him—if and when he deserves
it. It is here that the system founders. Most peer review
committees are reluctant to discipline physicians. A few
hospitals have even been sued by doctors who have been
deprived of their hospital privileges through disciplinary action of a peer review committee. These men sue for loss of
income and usually they win their cases. So today, the threat
of a suit by a doctor disciplined by a peer review committee
is enough to make that committee back down. Dr. Frances
Norris, a Washington D.C. pathologist, has put it this way:
"They [the committee] have no real power to discipline offenders nor any way to protect themselves from lawsuits that
may be brought against them." More than any group in the
world, doctors and hospitals have a horror of publicity and
will take almost any evasive action to stay out of the lime-
light. Too many peer review committees in community hospitals are controlled by the chiefs of the sections of surgery
and medicine. These men, as we have seen, are all too often

the worst offenders themselves in performing unnecessary operations and demanding laboratory tests and X-rays so they are in no position to control and police others. It is no accident that the chiefs of the various services are the highest earners in the medical profession, and they tend to maintain the status quo as long as other physicians do not question their activities or are willing to toe the line. Unfortunately members of a peer review committee are not likely to be tough on colleagues whom they see every day in the hospital staff room or whose wives play bridge and tennis together. They are also reluctant to crack the whip over someone on whom they depend for referrals. Rotating the membership of the peer review committee has been proposed as an answer to these problems, but experience has shown that the reaction is not to bear down too heavily on a man who next month will be reviewing *your* work.

Such problems have led physicians like Dr. Norris to declare that "internal regulatory committees of hospitals are by and large non-functioning figureheads." Dr. Lowell E. Bellin, New York City's first deputy commissioner of health, agrees. "Peer review within a single hospital is a clear conflict of interest," he told Senator Edward M. Kennedy (D. Mass.) during Congressional hearings on the health care crisis in America. At the very least, one hospital should review the work of another, Dr. Bellin maintained.

Peer review works best where it is needed least, it was pointed out in a recent article on the subject in the physicians' news magazine, *Medical World News.* In a first-rate hospital, where good physicians are most likely to be found devoting themselves to raising standards that are already high, peer review gives added confidence in the way the patients are managed.

But in a poorly run hospital, where there is by definition room for improvement, the staff tends simply to go through the motions of reviewing cases. The situation is even worse where the hospital is a proprietary institution being run for profit. Here the review committee's criterion is most likely to be whether or not the work done was profitable, not whether it was justified. If the review committee recommended a course that could interfere with profits, the management would be likely to overrule them.

Yet another problem with peer review is that it is like locking the door after the horse is stolen. What is the use of reviewing the activities of the medical staff if the patient is already dead or permanently crippled? The increasing number of medical malpractice suits is evidence of the public's awareness of and concern over uneven medical services. If a peer review board prevents future patients from exposure to incompetent physicians, then it is serving a useful purpose. But would it not be better to prevent the incompetent man from practicing in the first place?

So, to the consumer or patient, peer review has only an indirect benefit. Certainly it is comforting for a sick person to know that the hospital care he is receiving is subject to objective evaluation, but he will never know—nor can he ever find out—how his own doctor's work is rated by his colleagues. There is nothing in the medical profession like the Better Business Bureau, where complaints are registered and kept on file, and where these can be checked by the public. There is not even any such group as the Consumers' Union or Consumer Research to make unbiased comparisons of different products or procedures.

Some medical men have gone on record that the public ought to be represented on peer review boards—but usually

by "the public" they mean a banker or accountant who will
help to curb high fees. They are not talking about good medical care as such. So this attitude is only good as far as it
goes. Should the patient not also be able to learn from some
authoritative body whether or not everything possible has
been done in their case? And if not—why not?

To date, there is no satisfactory answer to this natural
query.

XVI

Quality Control of Medical Care
—Some New Proposals

1. *Federal Inspection of Medicine*
U.S. INDICTS SURGEON
FOR POOR PRACTICE
WASHINGTON, D.C.—The Justice Department today charged a surgeon with doing too much surgery. The indictment was handed down in Federal District Court following an investigation of the surgeon's activities. The charge is the first to be brought under a new law, recently passed by Congress, which set up a system to control unwarranted surgery and medical care. . . .

The above newspaper story is a fiction. No law exists today under which a doctor can be accused of doing excessive surgery. But it may well become fact in the not-too-distant future. If such a law is passed, it could mean greater protection for the patient against excessive medical attention —and better overall care.

Senator Edward Kennedy has proposed the most comprehensive of the various national health insurance proposals

155

currently before Congress. And it has probably the most far-reaching implications for the future of the American medical care. If passed in its present form, it could bring the standards of American health delivery up to those of other industrially advanced countries which already have such services.

However, no health insurance plan, not even Kennedy's, spells out any definite guidelines on providing proper controls over the medical profession. None of the proposed legislation would prevent the kinds of abuses discussed in this book. Doctors would still be free to engage in questionable or unnecessary treatment.

Senator Kennedy has suggested that there may be federal control of the medical profession some day. He has said, at his hearings on the health care crisis in America, that if his national health insurance bill should become law, it would be given a set of regulatory teeth to control the overall-treatment of patients.

The consumer might even be worse off with national health insurance legislation as it is presently drafted, because, like the Medicare and Medicaid plans, it would give physicians and hospitals open access to the public purse, letting them dip into it virtually at will. The result could be a continuation of the increasing costs of health without any guarantee that the patient would be getting improved care.

Any improvement in the present health delivery system that sets out to provide basic universal care must be coupled with far more rigid quality controls than are prevailing at present or being suggested. Our experience with Medicare and Medicaid has shown that a government-backed health insurance system cannot be left in the hands of the medical profession or hospital administrators without outside supervision. To paraphrase the French statesman Georges Briand: "Medicine is too important a thing to leave to the physicians."

In order to regulate and control the "activities" of physicians and hospitals the following specific proposals are offered.

What is needed is a federal system of quality control of medical services that is free of influence by local pressure groups—such as doctors controlling the governing boards of their own local hospitals. This includes the chiefs of the various hospital services such as medicine and surgery. The Department of Health Education and Welfare (HEW) should be empowered to set up and operate the system, employing on a full-time basis, a corps of physicians trained in the various medical and surgical specialties; radiology, anesthesia, pathology, laboratory services, and hospital administration.

These experts, both the medically trained and those experienced in health-care delivery, would serve as inspectors of all medical services whether these were paid for by national health insurance, or through semi-public plans like Blue Cross and Blue Shield, or by private insurance plans, or even directly by the patient.

These federally appointed inspectors should function like the professional auditors employed by the Internal Revenue Service. They would be assigned to go around the country examining all hospital and physician records. While they would review reports made by existing peer review groups, they would not necessarily be influenced by them. Every physician's records would be reviewed, including those of the various chiefs of medical and surgical services, since they frequently are the worse offenders and set the tone for others to follow.

The inspectors would come to an independent judgment concerning the quality of the care that was being provided and whether or not it was necessary from the recorded facts in the case reports. They would also be empowered to request the physician and other members of the health care team to provide additional information on any case that seemed to require it.

To assure that these inspectors conducted themselves with complete impartiality, it would be necessary to see that they did not become influenced by local medical politicians or hierarchies. This would mean rotating these inspectors periodically to different territories of the country.

About twice a year, the work of every physician, no matter what his practice or specialty, should be reviewed by an inspector who would, of course, be fully qualified in the particular specialty of the physician whose work he was studying. The inspector would then make a report to HEW. If, in his opinion, there were instances of unnecessary medical care, surgery, or of poor medical practice, the physician concerned would be interviewed privately so that both he and the inspector had a clear understanding of the reasons for the adverse report. The type of things that would be covered would be, for instance, the treatment of cases outside of the physicians specialty—particularly surgery—excessive attention on some cases to the possible neglect of others, too many tonsillectomes, hysterectomies, cholecystectomies and the like, possibly even the need of the doctor to retire or to cut down active practice due to his own health problems.

When HEW received a critical report on a doctor, it would be empowered to issue him a warning. If, on the next inspection, the irregularities in his practice continued, he could be fined in accordance with a declared scale. If the abuses went on after that, legal proceedings could be taken against him. He would of course have the right of appeal against adverse judgment as in any other forms of federal regulation.

According to the American Medical Association figures, there are approximately 300,000 licensed physicians in the United States. Of these a little over 30 percent are full-time salaried men: teachers in medical schools, physicians in the Armed Forces, Veterans Administration, state and city hospitals, as well as residents and interns. This leaves some 200,000 physicians who practice medicine and surgery on some sort of fee-for-service basis. Assuming each inspector hired by HEW for quality control purposes could study the work of two doctors each week, one inspector could review about a hundred doctors a year.

This would involve hiring a corps of some two to three thousand physician-inspectors in various specialties. Assuming they were paid, in round figures, a salary of $30,000 a year, and allowing $10,000 for expenses per inspector and $10,000 per year for clerical and secretarial assistance, the total cost of such a system of 3,000 inspectors might amount to around $150 million a year, including federal inspectors for hospital services.

This is only 0.2 percent of the estimated $70 billion annual cost of the national health insurance plan proposed by Senator Kennedy.

Furthermore, the cost of operating this quality control system would be offset for the taxpayer by substantially reducing the number of hospitalizations, drugs, and laboratory and X-ray tests, etc., prescribed by doctors. It might well drop by half the number of unnecessary elective surgical procedures performed nowadays, while considerably reduc-

ing the number of operations for hernia repair, hemor-
rhoidectomies or varicose veins. Similar reductions in other
branches of medical practice might also be expected.

These savings could in turn be redistributed to the disadvantaged and those who now receive very inadequate medical care—as well as to those who are genuinely sick. The
mechanism would provide adequate universal health care
without any substantial increase in costs above present
levels.

The inclusion of those now medically disadvantaged into
the health care system as a whole would mean that there
would be no shrinkage in the health industry or sudden unemployment in medical ranks. Hospital beds would still be
occupied but by really sick people. The present structure of
health care delivery would continue as before.

The only change would be that those who today are being
over-treated would be replaced by those who really need
treatment. This could improve working conditions for the
medical profession as a whole since specialists would not
have to be constantly seeking out patients from referring
physicians in order to keep themselves occupied and their
earnings on the increase.

A long-range advantage from such a review system would
be the automatic collection of information on patterns of
disease and the best methods of managing it. There would
be, in the files of HEW's inspectors, a dynamic picture of
the natural history of illnesses that could help in the evolu-
tion of effective treatment and its modification where needed. This could make for a more meaningful use of our health
services, since we would have some idea of the advantages in
not doing a medical or surgical procedure as opposed to actually doing it. At the moment no such clearing house of in-

formation exists on such a broad scale.

There should be no particular difficulty in recruiting inspectors for a Federal Medical Inspection System. Many well-qualified men and women in the various specialities who originally went into the profession because of their dedication to healing would welcome the opportunity to be of real service in this way. Every year, the U.S. Public Health Service recruits sizeable numbers of full-time younger doctors to work in state and federal health agencies or clinical research laboratories such as those supported by the National Institutes of Health. Further, there is a surplus of young, bright, well-trained men in various specialities of medicine and surgery, hanging around the fringes of medical schools, waiting for a position of challenge, who would welcome such an opportunity. Also some middle-aged physicians who wish to retire from active private practice because of some physical illness may take up such jobs.

They would be men (and women) of unquestionable qualifications and training and with the academic background to examine critically and constructively the medical activities of the physicians inspected. Such individuals should be board certified in the various specialties that they would review. It is believed that they would be able to enforce better quality control of medical practice than that of the present system of "peer review."

2. Patient "Needs" versus "Wants"

What a patient needs and what a patient or his physician wants in terms of medical care should be clearly separated. The term *need* should refer to a person who is acutely ill with some known or unknown disease requiring immediate hospitalization and treatment. The term *want* should refer to elective surgery, medical "checkup" or treatment desired by the patient or his physician for largely imagined illnesses.

An example of "need" would be following accidental injury, a person with an acute pain in the abdomen, with a suspicion of appendicitis or a strangulated hernia, or a patient with an acute chest pain with a possibility of coronary thrombosis, or a person who is acutely short of breath with some acute respiratory difficulty.

"Want" would include elective surgery such as treatment to correct minor physical problems like wens, warts, hernias, varicose veins, or plastic and cosmetic surgery. It would also include the giving of unnecessary laboratory tests and X-rays for possibly undiagnosed diseases—so called "check-ups."

The people who "need" hospitalization or acute medical and surgical therapy obviously should be taken care of first, and the government and third party insurance should cover the cost of these illnesses completely. The "wanted" surgery and tests could be paid for separately, either directly by the individual or through specially bought insurance programs designed to specifically cover this type of treatment.

The medical educators should be asked to clearly define the various disease processes constituting the two categories. The federal inspectors should then enforce this classification on physicians, hospitals and nursing homes. (This is, in essence, the way the National Health Service operates in Great Britain.)

3. Fee Schedules for Various Medical Conditions

A uniform fee schedule should be developed for managing specific diseases. For example, if a patient has pneumonia, a physician would be paid a certain fee. This fee would be fixed throughout the country. This fee would be the same regardless of the number of days of hospitalization or the number of laboratory tests or X-rays performed, although, of course, it would take into account that some period of hospitalization and some laboratory work may be necessary. However, by instituting such a fixed-fee schedule relative to the disease in question, a considerable number of unnecessarily long hospital stays, and unnecessary laboratory studies could be eliminated. Many studies, if needed in the opinion of the physician attending the case, could be done in the doctor's office or in the out-patient services of the laboratory or hospital clinic. Similar schedules of fees should be developed for hospitals to be paid according to various disease processes, rather than according to the number of hospital days, laboratory tests or X-rays performed.

A parallel situation already exists in surgery. A surgeon, when he does an "exploratory operation" as opposed to a definitive surgical procedure, does not get paid for the full procedure, only a fee for the "exploratory." Most surgeons, today, have to abide by fee schedules set for well-defined operative procedures. This system could now be applied to medical care for suspected although unproven diseases, for instance "heart attacks" that turn out to be only false alarms in 50 percent of the cases. Similarly, fee schedules could be applied to roentgenologists, pathologists, and anaesthesiologists for their respective services, according to disease.

Similar fixed-payment schedules could be developed for the hospitals, clinics and nursing homes rather than, as at present, for the number of hospital days, laboratory tests or X-rays performed. This would help to eliminate unncessary laboratory tests and prolonged hospitalization.

4. Foster Homes for the Aged

The cost of nursing homes has risen with the cost of hospitalization. An average nursing home costs from $30 to $35 a day. To help reduce this cost, setting up a system of "foster homes" is suggested for marginally ill patients requiring minimal nursing care, who are not completely incapacitated, but who have no family able or willing to take care of them. By providing such foster homes, one could put the patients into a home environment where he (or she) would be happier than in an institution. The family caring for such individuals would of course be paid for the service but it probably could be provided at half the price paid to a nursing home. Patients would still be under the care of their own physicians.

These foster homes could be provided by retired couples with homes larger than they need to supplement their income and who are healthy enough to care for someone who needs only the most routine nursing care. It is possible that many retired nurses would like to take in one or two such patients into their own homes. The idea would be to provide the patients with a home environment that is emotionally and psychologically more fulfilling than being placed into institutional "waiting rooms for death." These foster homes would, of course, be inspected for proper quality control by the same authorities who inspect regular nursing homes. Of course patients requiring special nursing care for terminal illnesses would still be treated in nursing homes.

Some agencies, such as the Family and Child Services of Washington, D.C., are already operating such foster homes systems for the elderly, on a small scale.

5. No Fault Insurance

A "no fault insurance" plan to control the rising number of medical malpractice suits is suggested. In this system, a voluntary pool of money would be created by physicians, hospitals and nursing homes through insurance premiums. Any claims or injuries arising out of alleged improper care of patients by the physicians, hospitals, or nursing homes would be referred to an impartial panel or board which, on the basis of the evidence available, would decide on the extent of the injury suffered by the claimant and then award the claimant the appropriate amount they considered commensurate with the injuries suffered. The awards would be made on the basis of a "no fault" system similar to the new Massachusetts automobile insurance system.

Every patient, upon admission to hospital, would sign an agreement to accept the board's decision on any compensation for accidental injuries sustained during hospitalization, similar to the awards made by the Industrial Accident and Workman's Compensation Act. This would not necessarily preclude any future action for deliberate criminal negligence or action on the part of the physician, hospital, nursing home or their agents. It would leave the patient free to request a district attorney's investigation of any deliberate or criminal wrong-doing or free to sue for damages sustained.

With this sort of insurance program, it is believed that there would be a reduction in the many so-called "nuisance" law suits. The arbitration panel's decisions would be on the basis of injuries sustained and the compensation necessary, not on the basis of the "deepest pocket" principle. This would free both the doctors as well as the hospitals from performing unnecessary hospitalizations, laboratory tests and X-rays to protect themselves against the possibility of malpractice suits, as well as lower the cost of malpractice insurance premiums, which ultimately the consumer pays.

While such a concept has many proponents—both in and out of medicine—it is only fair to add that it may not completely solve the problem of adequately compensating patients injured by medical and surgical treatment.

For injuries resulting from clear-cut cases of mis-management, a no-fault system might work well, but unfortunately most injuries are not that simple. A leading physician who is also an attorney, Dr. Don Harper Mills of the University of Southern California, has pointed out that if a no-fault system were to compensate for every injury as a result of medical and surgical management, then the end result could possibly even increase the premiums paid by doctors for coverage against malpractice. This in turn would force up the patient's medical bill even higher.

For example, a patient with an acute appendix which burst, causing peritonitis and eventual death is described by Dr. Mills. If this patient had sought medical advice in time and surgery was unduly delayed for insufficient reason, then the doctor might indeed be liable under present law.

But suppose an appendix ruptures, or suppose a patient delays or refuses surgery. Then, according to Dr. Mills, the doctor is clearly not at fault and, under the present system of determining liability in the courts, he could successfully defend himself. Under a no fault system, however, compensation for the untoward result of a burst appendix might be paid without question. If this happened with any regularity, the cost of malpractice insurance to cover the cost of such claims would be overwhelming.

To avoid this type of situation, Dr. Mills suggests a more limited type of coverage—one that would only pay for injuries actually caused by medical or surgical mistakes—no matter whether the mistake was the result of negligence or not. Unfortunately, he believes that almost as much time and effort would be needed to ascertain whether such mistakes were really the cause of the patient's·injury as is at present spent in legal proceedings to determine who is at fault.

6. Specialist Fees for Specialist Work

As noted earlier, there are many physicians who designate themselves as specialists and are in fact not certified as such by any recognized specialty board. Despite this, such individuals charge specialist fees, and insurance carriers, including the federal government, pay such fees without question. This is a clear misrepresentation on the part of the physician that must amount to several billion dollars in the course of a year. No matter who pays such "specialists," it all adds to our already inflated national medical bill.

Therefore, we propose that health insurance carriers should be required to check up on the credentials of the specialists through the *Directory of Medical Specialists* and only pay specialist fees to various specialty board-certified men. There is really no reason for either the government controlled plans such as Medicare and Medicaid or the private health insurors to make payments to self-designated specialists who are really "non-specialists." This move will increase the ranks of general practitioners, so badly needed.

The adoption of this policy, probably one of the simplest moves that could currently be made to reduce medical costs, would not only result in a direct saving on individual medical bills, but would eliminate the necessity for redoing the bad jobs done on patients by unqualified men. The result would be a general improvement in the quality of surgical and medical specialist procedures. It might even reduce the number of malpractice suits—which currently run to $100 million a year and up—against physicians and hospitals. This in turn would reduce the risk of malpractice and therefore the size of malpractice insurance premiums—the cost of which ultimately are reflected in the patient's bill.

7. *Control of Those Entering the Specialties*

As noted earlier, many more young doctors train for the surgical specialty than for any other medical specialty. This has led to serious incongruities in proper medical care. For example, few operations can be performed without general anesthesia, yet while there are more than 75,000 surgeons in the U.S. there are less than 10,000 anesthesiologists, resulting in improperly trained doctors and nurses administering anaesthesia, with greater danger to the patients. Maybe, as Dr. John Bunker of Stanford University Medical School in Palo Alto, California, has suggested, this means that there are not enough anesthesiologists. However, might it not also mean, he pointed out, that there are too many surgeons? Health maintainance organizations like Kaiser Permanente Group require only six general surgeons per 100,000 persons under a prepaid plan, while under the usual fee-for-service system the nation at large "uses" thirteen surgeons per 100,000 persons.

Whatever the reason, you, the patient, are badly served because no matter how good the surgery is, if the anaesthetic is not correctly administered, you could easily suffer permanent injury or even death.

We suggest, therefore, that there should be some overall system of control over the numbers of physicians training in the various medical and surgical specialties. The figure at any one time of those in training should be based on the actual need for that particular specialty in the light of medical care nationwide. In other words, there should be some central agency in HEW through which the nationwide needs for various specialists could be projected. The rates at which these specialists are being trained could be adjusted accordingly. The data for such requirements can be collected from local and national medical societies, from city, and state and federal health agencies, and, last but not least, from the findings of the federal medical inspecjors. Such "control" will be resisted vociferously, but, in actuality, it is no more than the reasonable management of limited human resources that is exercised by the medical services of the Armed Forces.

It is estimated that by legislative adoption and executive enforcement of these proposals at least a reduction by half in the cost of the present health care budget can be obtained. The savings thus achieved can be used to finance the health needs of all Americans regardless of their socio-economic status.

The physicians and hospitals would then be serving all truly sick people, rather than engaging in excessive and frequently unnecessary care of a few. This optimal level of health care can be achieved without causing any economic discomfort to the related health industry or health personnel. They would continue to find employment, health care facilities would spread to those 30 million "other Americans" who are at present largely neglected because of the combined crippling affect of poverty, unemployment, or minority status.

Epilogue

When Dr. Milford O. Rouse, a Dallas gastroenterologist, declared in 1967, as president of the American Medical Association, that he believed medical care was a privilege and not a right, he set off a hare that with no signs of fatigue has been breasting the uplands ever since, hotly pursued by a motley gathering of emphysematous physicians, health care economists, and outspoken members of the public—all in states of mind ranging from outright agreement with Dr. Rouse to sheer outrage.

Listening to the various arguments may be entertaining, but it is hardly enlightening. Dr. Rouse and his debators miss the point. It is not whether health care is a right or a privilege that is at issue—it is whether we can afford to have a significant part of the population in poor health and still remain a viable community. It is clear that we cannot.

Poor health cripples a society just as surely as it does an individual, and we can no longer afford to have our medical resources (which are and will always be limited) devoted to over-caring for one group in our country at the expense of another.

There are many aspects of our present crisis in medical and health services that we have not been able to mention or adequately discuss due to lack of space. Sufficient to repeat that millions of our fellow citizens (whose lives impinge on our own) daily face stark tragedy and bumbling confusion in our health care delivery system. Self-respecting middle-class families have been brought to bankruptcy by crushing medical bills. The poor and near-poor, who tend to have poorer health than the well-salaried and well-insured, find that medical care is almost unattainable. When they do find it, in order to receive it they have to survive humiliation and indifference of a kind that would deter many of us who were less urgently in need.

One answer to the problem is a reordering of medical priorities. These are genuine medical needs which the hospital and the medical community should deliver—quite apart from how they are paid for. These needs must be provided for because we cannot afford not to provide for them. Only after these needs are met should the medical community concern itself with treatments that are simply patients' desires.

Such things as selective surgery and treatments that represent patients' desires or wants should be paid for at the patient's own expense or through private insurance. They should certainly not be covered by any compulsory health insurance plan.

A system that clearly differentiates needs from desires (or wants) could, if well implemented, prevent much of the over-use of medical services by the well-to-do and free these services for those who at present receive inadequate health care or none at all.

171

A redistribution of medical facilities would not raise the cost of the nation's health bill by a cent and yet we would all, as a society, be healthier as a result. Wilbur Cohen, former secretary of the Department of Health, Education, and Welfare, has noted that health care is a public utility, subject to the same kinds of policy constraints that are exercised over other public utilities.

Present-day medical facilities have expanded to fill demands rather than demonstrable needs. No matter how medical services are to be organized in the future—to insure better medical care for yourself, use medical services only when you need them and then as little as possible.

This is, of course, an over-simplification of a very complex problem. There are many demonstrable needs in health which at present are not being met at all, and worse, show no signs of being met. Certainly there are times when one should use medical services even when one is not sick; regular checkups and other preventive measures pay off in the long run.

But, as we have tried to emphasize throughout this book, it is wrong to subject yourself and your family to over-care, and to guard against this, you must question your doctor about everything. Double-check, if you are not sure. Get an independent opinion before you undergo *any* surgery. Take drugs with only the greatest of caution and *only* as your doctor prescribes.

If need be, alter your life-style so that your health is maintained and improved. Cut risks to a minimum. All life consists of taking chances, but some chances are more necessary than others. Calculate the risks and act accordingly. That is what insurance companies do. It protects them as well as their customers.

Never forget that if you have a steady income and health insurance you represent a ripe plum to certain less-than-scrupulous medical men who, in the name of good medicine, adhere to the highwayman's motto: "Your money or your life!"

We have tried to provide an introductory guide that we hope will help you avoid illness, purchase medical care intelligently, and above all avoid the chicanery and deception that is practiced by some members of the medical profession. If you know enough to buy the best, you will recognize how to avoid the worst. Further, if you buy only the best, you will effectively put the bad elements of medicine out of business. This will not only help you, it will help us all.

This book was conceived and written in anguish at the way physicians have allowed certain of their fellows to debase a noble profession. It is also a warning to that profession as a whole that if they do not vigorously, effectively, and universally practice high standards and exercise concern for their patients, then they will have discarded a tradition of public service that goes back to the dawn of civilization. If the doctors do not act to put their own house in order, they may reverse the progress of medicine to the detriment not just of themselves but of all of society. The art and science of medical practice is not exclusive to the physicians, it belongs to us all. It is for the service of us all.

The physician, by virtue of his training, has accepted the responsibility of trust for the care and nurture of his chosen profession. If he continues to pursue a course of narrow self-interest, then he will find that he is no longer honored with this trust. The public will look elsewhere for the defence of its health, and the loss will be not only the doctor's but that of all men.

Although we have tried to indicate how the patient can ensure his own protection from unscrupulous members of the medical profession and how certain outside authorities could intervene to ensure this protection, such safeguards cannot take the place of the doctor's individual conscience and his sense of professional ethics.

The medical profession has to realize that the public has had enough. People are angry at the inadequate way they are currently being served by the medical and health professionals in this country, and they will not long continue to submit.

Some Recommended Reading

In recent years we have all become what is loosely called consumer oriented, although of course we have always been consumers—ever since primitive man swapped a cow for a wife with both the cow-owner and woman-owner hoping to gain by the trade. Equally, we have not always gained unless we weighed the transaction carefully.

Two thousand years before Ralph Nader, the Romans had a phrase for it which, despite the far more complex world of today, still holds good. "Caveat emptor"—Let the buyer beware—they said.

When it comes to purchasing or doing business, this principle is still valid, and nowhere more valid than in the purchase of medical care with its, ultimately, individual face-to-face relationship between the physician and his patient.

Applying the principle of caveat emptor, the knowledgeable buyer will not only help himself, he will even help others. If the purchaser of medical care insists on quality, and questions wasteful expenditures, he will improve the service he gets far more rapidly and efficiently than by depending on government and the legislative processes to do so.

175

It takes a little work to be knowledgeable about the purchase of your medical care, but it can be done without difficulty. The following list of books include some standard reference volumes that will be useful over the years. The others represent a very small cross-selection of the currently available books and reports that deal with today's problems.

FOR THE PERMANENT REFERENCE SHELF

1. A good medical dictionary, *Dorland*'s or *Stedman*'s. These are obtainable in any bookstore. Be sure you get the latest edition.

2. A sound up-to-date health guide. There are several published every year and new editions of old ones keep appearing. Aimed at the nonmedical reader, they can be bought at any bookstore. In general, these popular health guides provide useful information. Their main problem is their rather bland tone. One supposes that this is meant to be reassuring. a sort of literary version of the bedside manner, since most are written, edited, or at least supervised by medical men. Unfortunately the result is that their discussions lack fire and sometimes even reality, and therefore can be misleading.

3. *The Merck Manual*, obtainable from Information Service Manager, Merck Inc., Rahway, N.J. This is an excellent though highly technical compendium and is better than the standard medical textbooks that are expensive and, in today's rapidly changing world of medicine, often out of date. The *Manual* is written for the physician, not the layman, so you may have some difficulty at first. But persevere. With the aid of a good medical dictionary, you will find it contains much enlightening information on specific diseases. All in all, it is a very handy shield against poor doctoring. The book is revised regularly and is currently in its twelfth

edition. Be sure you get the latest one.

FOR BACKGROUND READING

Heal Yourself: Report of the Citizens Board of Inquiry into Health Services for Americans is obtainable from the American Public Health Association, 1015 18th Street N. W. Washington, D. C. 20036.

This challenging paper describes our health services in terms of the personal experiences of Americans in many walks of life. It illustrates what is wrong with our health services and describes several efforts that have been made by dedicated physicians with varying degress of success, to improve them. The report loses nothing by including a minority dissenting opinion that reflects in microcosm the current debate among physicians and health professionals concerning the organization and provision of good medical care for all.

Health Care in Transition: Directions for the Future by Anne R. Somers. Hospital Research and Education Trust, 840 Lake Shore Drive, Chicago, Ill. 60611.

Mrs. Somers' book is a pleasant exception to much of the authoritative writing on medical and health economics. Doctors are often criticized for their poor writing and not entirely without foundation. But compared with the impenetrable prose of most of the experts on the economics of health care, they are models of clarity.

Here is an excellent and up-to-date summary of the present state of our health system and how it got the way it is, why it does the things it does, and doesn't do the things it should. It's a fine primer to help you prepare yourself for the coming debates on national health insurance and the form this should eventually take. Mrs. Somers will help you clarify your thinking about how to achieve the best kind of health care for the American people.

FOR GENERAL READING

How to Avoid Unnecessary Surgery by Lawrence P. Williams, M.D., Nash Publishing, Los Angeles.

This is an excellent guidebook for the patient faced with the possibility of a surgical operation. To go under the knife or not? That is Dr. Williams' question and he tends to answer in the negative.

Clearly and succintly he details the risks of operating in a number of common surgical procedures and provides a useful, although not exhaustive, summary of the general background the patient needs to make an intelligent decision. One nice touch is that Dr. Williams practices what he preaches and in so doing has managed to avoid a great deal of surgery recommended at various times for himself and his family. This is a very valuable consumer's guide to one aspect of medicine.

Five Patients: The Hospital Explained, by Michael Crichton, M.D., Bantam Books.

This is a splendid account of what happens to a patient when he comes under the care of a modern, urban, teaching hospital. Using the experiences of five patients admitted to Massachusetts General Hospital in Boston as an illustration, Dr. Crichton weaves a fascinating web showing up-to-date hospital medicine at work. You will come away from this book with a much greater understanding of physicians and their problems as you see them trying to help patients with theirs.

Dr. Crichton fills in his case reports with an informative historical perspective that explains much about why medicine is practiced the way it is. Such an understanding is essential if we are ever to improve our health services. Too few of today's critics of medicine have this understanding.

One word of warning, however, and it comes from Dr. Crichton himself. There is nothing typical about either the patients whose experiences he describes or the hospital where they were treated. In short, he presents some examples of what must be nearly the best in medical care for the acutely ill anywhere in the world. Therefore by definition, Dr. Crichton's five patients are special cases. And, even if their experiences were typical of hospitals in general, care of the acutely ill is only a part of what we need in health and medical services.

In Critical Condition: The Crisis in America's Health Care by Edward M. Kennedy, Simon and Schuster.

In the spring of 1971, the Democratic senator from Massachusetts held a series of public hearings around the country as well as in Washington on the health care crisis in the United States. Before him paraded a long line of expert and not-so-expert witnesses who testified, some in highly moving terms, on the desperate state they had been reduced to by their brush with one or another aspect of the medical profession and its ancillary services. This book is largely a boiled-down version of the testimony with, of course, Senator Kennedy's prescription for the ailing health care system —his own national health insurance proposal.

If you are in any doubt that our medical care system is in need of revision, this book provides a useful corrective. But, as presented here, the Senator's therapeutic measures are inadequate to managing the criticial condition in which he finds his patient.

Index